Treating Fear of Cancer Recurrence
with Group Cognitive-Behavioural Therapy:
A Step-by-Step Guide

Josée Savard • Aude Caplette-Gingras
Lucie Casault • Jennifer Hains

Treating Fear of Cancer Recurrence with Group Cognitive-Behavioural Therapy: A Step-by-Step Guide

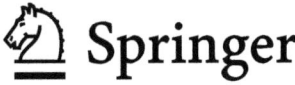

Josée Savard
School of Psychology, Université Laval
CHU de Québec-Université Laval
Research Center
Québec, QC, Canada

Lucie Casault
Department of Multidisciplinary Services
CHU de Québec-Université Laval
Québec, QC, Canada

Aude Caplette-Gingras
Hôpital du St-Sacrement, CHU de Québec-Université Laval
CHU de Québec-Université Laval
Research Center
Québec, QC, Canada

Jennifer Hains
CHU de Québec-Université Laval
Québec, QC, Canada

ISBN 978-3-031-07189-8   ISBN 978-3-031-07187-4 (eBook)
https://doi.org/10.1007/978-3-031-07187-4

© The Editor(s) (if applicable) and The Author(s), under exclusive license to Springer Nature Switzerland AG 2022
This work is subject to copyright. All rights are solely and exclusively licensed by the Publisher, whether the whole or part of the material is concerned, specifically the rights of reprinting, reuse of illustrations, recitation, broadcasting, reproduction on microfilms or in any other physical way, and transmission or information storage and retrieval, electronic adaptation, computer software, or by similar or dissimilar methodology now known or hereafter developed.
The use of general descriptive names, registered names, trademarks, service marks, etc. in this publication does not imply, even in the absence of a specific statement, that such names are exempt from the relevant protective laws and regulations and therefore free for general use.
The publisher, the authors and the editors are safe to assume that the advice and information in this book are believed to be true and accurate at the date of publication. Neither the publisher nor the authors or the editors give a warranty, expressed or implied, with respect to the material contained herein or for any errors or omissions that may have been made. The publisher remains neutral with regard to jurisdictional claims in published maps and institutional affiliations.

This Springer imprint is published by the registered company Springer Nature Switzerland AG
The registered company address is: Gewerbestrasse 11, 6330 Cham, Switzerland

We would like to dedicate this book to our beloved children Clément, Estelle, Eva, Hugo, Nellie, Laurier, Olivier, and Romy.

Acknowledgments

The writing of this manual would not have been possible without the significant contribution of others to whom we wish to convey our warmest thanks.

First of all, we would like to express our gratitude to all the patients who participated in our psychotherapy groups focusing on fear of cancer recurrence. Their involvement, the medical and personal experiences they shared, and their constructive comments have enabled us to continuously improve the program.

We would also like to thank our fellow psychologists specialized in oncology at the CHU de Québec-Université Laval. Exchanging views with you on the content of the program was extremely helpful. Also, a big thank you to our graduate students and interns in psychology who observed and co-animated the psychotherapy groups. Teaching them the rationale for the interventions and how to use them allowed us to refine our ideas for this book which we hope will be useful in helping more patients dealing with fear of cancer recurrence. More particulary, we want to recognize the contribution of Marie-Hélène Savard, Véronique Massicotte, Catherine Banville and Catherine Filion.

Finally, we would like to thank Humanov-is, who helped us structure the training program to administer this psychotherapy, Université Laval for funding our dissemination efforts through a social innovation research program , and Mélanie Dixon who worked on the translation of the book.

Contents

Part I   Psychotherapy Group on Fear of Cancer Recurrence: Therapist's Manual

1 Session No. 1 3
- 1.1 Introduction 4
  - 1.1.1 Slide #1: Fear of Cancer Recurrence 4
  - 1.1.2 Slide #2: Psychotherapy Group on Fear of Cancer Recurrence 5
  - 1.1.3 Slide #3: Warning 7
- 1.2 Content of the Sessions 8
  - 1.2.1 Slide #4: Content of the Sessions 8
  - 1.2.2 Slide #5: Session No. 1 9
- 1.3 Information on Fear of Cancer Recurrence 10
  - 1.3.1 Slide #6: Fear of Cancer Recurrence 11
  - 1.3.2 Slide #7: The Vicious Circle of Fear of Recurrence ... 12
- 1.4 Beliefs About the Influence of Psychological Factors on Cancer 14
  - 1.4.1 Slide #8: The Vicious Circle of Fear of Recurrence ... 15
  - 1.4.2 Slide #9: The Power of Thought 16
  - 1.4.3 Slide #10: Influence of Psychological Factors on Cancer 17
  - 1.4.4 Slide #11: Popular Beliefs 18
  - 1.4.5 Slide #12: Clinical Cases vs. Scientific Research 19
- 1.5 Stress = Cancer? 20
  - 1.5.1 Slide #13: Stress → Cancer? 21
  - 1.5.2 Slide #14: Multifactorial Model of Cancer 24
- 1.6 Positive Thoughts = Cure? 25
  - 1.6.1 Slide #15: Mental Attitude and Cancer Survival – Study 1 26
  - 1.6.2 Slide #16: Mental Attitude and Cancer Survival – Study 2 27
  - 1.6.3 Slide #17: Why Is It Important to Let Go of These Beliefs? 28
  - 1.6.4 Slide #18: Summary 29

1.7	The Cognitive Model of Emotions	30
	1.7.1 Slide #19: Cancer: A Distressing Experience	31
	1.7.2 Slide #20: Cognitive Model of Emotions (Beck)	32
1.8	The Vicious Circle of the Tyranny of Positive Thinking: The Case of Melissa	33
	1.8.1 Slides #21–22: The Case of Melissa	33
	1.8.2 Slide #23: The Case of Melissa (Continued)	35
	1.8.3 Slide #24: The Tyranny of Positive Thinking	36
	1.8.4 Slide #25: Negative Thoughts vs. Positive Thoughts	37
	1.8.5 Slide #26: Effects of Positive Thinking	38
1.9	What Does Research Say About the Effects of Positive Thinking?	40
	1.9.1 Slide #27: Effects of Optimism	41
	1.9.2 Slide #28: Fighting Cancer?	42
1.10	The Benefits of Realistic Thinking	44
	1.10.1 Slide #29: Dark Glasses vs. Rose-Coloured Glasses	44
	1.10.2 Slide #30: Is There an Alternative?	45
	1.10.3 Slide #31: Realistic Thoughts or Clear Glasses	46
	1.10.4 Slide #32: What Is Realistic Thinking?	47
	1.10.5 Slides #33–34: The Case of Mary	48
	1.10.6 Slide #35: Mary and Realistic Thoughts	50
	1.10.7 Slide #36: Benefits of Realistic Thinking	52
	1.10.8 Slides #37–38: The Case of Louise	53
	1.10.9 Slide #39: Cancer and Realistic Thoughts	55
	1.10.10 Slide #40: Do You Need to Change Your Way of Seeing Things?	57
1.11	Cognitive-Behavioural Therapy	57
	1.11.1 Slide #41: Cognitive-Behavioural Therapy	58
1.12	Recognizing Negative Thoughts	59
	1.12.1 Slide #42: Characteristics of Negative Thoughts	59
1.13	Thought Identification Exercise	61
	1.13.1 Slide #43: Identification of Negative Thoughts	61
	1.13.2 Slide #44: Exercise to Do at Home	62
1.14	Slide #45: End of Session Discussion	63
1.15	Slide #46: Tools in Brief	64
References		64

2 Session No. 2 ... 67

2.1	Session Agenda	68
	2.1.1 Slide #3: Session No. 2	68
2.2	Review of the Previous Session	69
2.3	Review of Last Week's Exercise	70
	2.3.1 Slide #4: Review of the Thought Identification Exercise	70
2.4	Fear of Cancer Recurrence Model	71
	2.4.1 Slide #5: The Vicious Circle of Fear of Recurrence	71
2.5	Cognitive Restructuring	72

		2.5.1	Slide #6: Cognitive Restructuring Grid	72
		2.5.2	Slide #7: The Case of Elise	73
		2.5.3	Slide #8: Fear of Recurrence	74
		2.5.4	Slide #9: The Case of Elise	75
		2.5.5	Slide #10: Questioning Your Thoughts	76
		2.5.6	Slide #11: The Case of Elise	78
		2.5.7	Slide #12: Recurrence ≠ Death	80
	2.6	Interpreting Physical Symptoms..................................		81
		2.6.1	Slide #13: Interpreting Physical Symptoms Realistically...	81
		2.6.2	Slide #14: Interpreting Physical Symptoms Realistically (NILP)	83
	2.7	Information-Seeking Profiles		86
		2.7.1	Slide #15: The Importance of Seeking the Right Information	86
	2.8	Being Well Informed		89
		2.8.1	Slide #16: Being Well Informed	89
	2.9	Interpreting Probabilities and Statistics		91
		2.9.1	Slide #17: Interpreting Probabilities	92
		2.9.2	Slide #18: Interpreting Probabilities	93
		2.9.3	Slide #19: Interpreting Probabilities	94
		2.9.4	Slide #20: Interpreting Probabilities	95
		2.9.5	Slide #17: Interpreting Probabilities (Go Back to a Previous Slide)	95
	2.10	Cognitive Restructuring Exercise		98
		2.10.1	Slide #21: Exercise to Do at Home	98
		2.10.2	Slides # 22-23: Cognitive Restructuring Grid and Questionning your Thoughts	99
	2.11	Slide #24: End of Session Discussion		101
	2.12	Slide #25: Tools in Brief...		102
	References...			103
3	Session No. 3			105
	3.1	Session Agenda...		106
		3.1.1	Slide #3: Session No. 3	106
	3.2	Review of the Previous Session		107
	3.3	Review of Last Week's Exercise...................................		107
		3.3.1	Slide #4: A Look Back on Cognitive Restructuring	107
		3.3.2	Slide #5: Cognitive Restructuring Grid	108
		3.3.3	Slide #6: Questioning Your Thoughts	109
	3.4	Intolerance of Uncertainty		110
		3.4.1	Slide #7: The Vicious Circle of Fear of Recurrence	110
		3.4.2	Slide #8: Intolerance of Uncertainty	111
		3.4.3	Slide #9: What Do You Think of the Following Statements?...	114
		3.4.4	Slide #10: Learning to Tolerate Uncertainty	116

- 3.5 Erroneous Beliefs about Worry 117
  - 3.5.1 Slide #11: The Usefulness and Impact of Worrying 117
  - 3.5.2 Slide #12: Behavioural Experiment 120
  - 3.5.3 Slide #13: Summary...................................... 121
- 3.6 Behavioural Avoidance.. 122
  - 3.6.1 Slide #14: The Vicious Circle of Fear of Recurrence........ 123
  - 3.6.2 Slide #15: Avoidance 124
  - 3.6.3 Slide #16: Avoidance and Habituation Curves............. 125
  - 3.6.4 Slide #17: Behavioural Exposure Rules 127
  - 3.6.5 Slide #18: Avoidance and Cancer 128
- 3.7 Behavioural Exposure Exercise 132
  - 3.7.1 Slide #19: The Importance of Facing Your Fears 132
  - 3.7.2 Slide #20: Exercise to Do at Home 133
  - 3.7.3 Slide #21: Behavioural Exposure.......................... 134
- 3.8 End of Session Discussion 136
  - 3.8.1 Slide #22: End of Session Discussion 136
- 3.9 Slide #23: Tools in Brief 137

4 Session No. 4.. 139
- 4.1 Session Agenda... 141
  - 4.1.1 Slide #3: Session No. 4 141
- 4.2 Review of the Previous Session 142
- 4.3 Review of Last Week's Exercise.................................... 143
  - 4.3.1 Slide #4: Review of the Behavioural Exposure Exercise.... 143
  - 4.3.2 Slide #5: The Vicious Circle of Fear of Recurrence 144
- 4.4 Cognitive Avoidance.. 145
  - 4.4.1 Slide #6: Cognitive Avoidance - The Camel Exercise 145
  - 4.4.2 Slide #7: Cognitive Avoidance 149
  - 4.4.3 Slide #8: The Importance of Facing Your Thoughts 150
- 4.5 Strategies to Counter Cognitive Avoidance 151
  - 4.5.1 Slide #9: Cognitive Restructuring......................... 152
  - 4.5.2 Slide #10: Planned "Worry Time"......................... 153
  - 4.5.3 Slide #11: Tolerating Negative Thoughts and Emotions... 154
  - 4.5.4 Slide #12: Cognitive Exposure 157
  - 4.5.5 Slide #13: Avoidance and Habituation Curves............. 158
- 4.6 Seeking Reassurance.. 159
  - 4.6.1 Slides #14–15: The Vicious Circle of Fear of Recurrence and Reassurance Seeking: A Form of Avoidance 160
  - 4.6.2 Slide #16: Reassurance Behaviour Examples 161
  - 4.6.3 Slide #17: Reassurance: Yes, But to What Extent? 162
- 4.7 Seeking Control.. 163
  - 4.7.1 Slide #18: Seeking Control 164
  - 4.7.2 Slide #19: Seeking Control 165
- 4.8 What If Cancer Comes Back?...................................... 166
  - 4.8.1 Slide #20: What If Cancer Comes Back? 167
  - 4.8.2 Slide #21: Recurrence ≠ Death 168

4.9	Redefining Life Goals	170
	4.9.1 Slide #22: The Importance of Life Goals	170
	4.9.2 Slides #23–24: The Case of Alfred	173
	4.9.3 Slide #25: Redefining Life Goals (Step 1)	176
	4.9.4 Slide #26: Redefining Life Goals (Step 2)	177
	4.9.5 Slide #27: Avenues for Reflection	178
4.10	Slide #28: End of Session Discussion	179
4.11	Slide #29: Tools in Brief	180
4.12	General Review of the Psychotherapy Group	181
	4.12.1 Slide #30: Conclusion	181
Reference		182

Part II Psychotherapy Group on Fear of Cancer Recurrence: Participant's Manual

5 Session No. 1 185
  5.1 What Is Fear of Recurrence? 185
    5.1.1 Fear of Recurrence: Is It Normal or Not? 185
    5.1.2 Understanding the Vicious Circle of Fear
           of Recurrence 186
  5.2 Can Thoughts Influence Cancer? 188
    5.2.1 Beliefs About the Influence of Psychological
           Factors on Cancer 188
    5.2.2 Does Stress Cause Cancer? 189
    5.2.3 Does Thought Have the Power to Cure Cancer? 190
    5.2.4 Can Positive Thinking Help You Cope with Cancer? .. 192
  5.3 The Cognitive Model of Emotions 192
    5.3.1 Cancer: A Distressing Experience 192
    5.3.2 The Cognitive Model and Adjustment to Cancer ... 194
  5.4 The Benefits of Realistic Thinking 194
    5.4.1 The Tyranny of Positive Thinking 194
    5.4.2 Fighting Cancer? 196
    5.4.3 Dark, Rose-Coloured, or Clear Glasses? 196
    5.4.4 Realistic Thinking and Cancer 200
  In Summary 202
  References 202

6 Session No. 2 203
  6.1 Cognitive Restructuring 203
    6.1.1 Cognitive Restructuring 203
    6.1.2 Cognitive Restructuring and Fear of Cancer
           Recurrence 206
  6.2 Interpreting Physical Symptoms Realistically 209
    6.2.1 Seeking the Right Information on Your Condition .. 211
  6.3 Being Well Informed 212

	6.4	Interpreting Probabilities and Statistics	213
	In Summary		214
	Reference		215
7	**Session No. 3**		**217**
	7.1	Intolerance of Uncertainty	217
	7.2	Learning to Tolerate Uncertainty	217
	7.3	Erroneous Beliefs about Worry	218
	7.4	The Importance of Facing Your Fears	220
		7.4.1 Avoidance and Habituation	221
	7.5	Behavioural Avoidance and Cancer	222
	7.6	Behavioural Exposure	223
	In Summary		225
8	**Session No. 4**		**227**
	8.1	Cognitive Avoidance	227
	8.2	Facing Your Thoughts	228
		8.2.1 Cognitive Restructuring	228
		8.2.2 Planned "Worry Time"	229
		8.2.3 Tolerating Unpleasant Thoughts and Emotions	229
		8.2.4 Cognitive Exposure	230
	8.3	Seeking Reassurance	231
	8.4	Seeking Control	232
	8.5	What If Cancer Comes Back?	233
	8.6	Redefining Life Goals	235
	In Summary		238
	8.7	Conclusion	239
	References		239
Appendix			**241**
Index			**251**

About the Authors

Josée Savard, PhD, is a psychologist and full professor in the School of Psychology at Université Laval and a researcher at the CHU de Québec-Université Laval Research Center. Her research interests are centered on the psychological aspects of cancer, more particularly insomnia, depression, and fear of cancer recurrence. She has published in French a book for the wider public (*Faire face au cancer avec la pensée réaliste* [Facing cancer with realistic thinking], Flammarion Quebec) of which some of the content was adapted for this book. In 2020, she also co-edited the *Handbook of Sleep Disorders in Medical Conditions* (Elsevier), which was awarded the PROSE award of the Association of American Publishers for the best handbook in medicine and clinical science.

Aude Caplette-Gingras, PhD, is a psychologist and a scientist-practitioner specialized in psycho-oncology. She is also in charge of professional practices development in psychology at the CHU de Québec-Université Laval. She works at the breast cancer clinic of the CHU de Québec-Université Laval (Hôpital du St-Sacrement). She has accumulated 13 years of experience using CBT in this population for a wide range of psychological problems, including fear of cancer recurrence. She also trains psychology interns in psycho-oncology.

Lucie Casault, PhD, is a psychologist specialized in oncology. She is head of the Department of Multidisciplinary Services at the CHU de Québec-Université Laval (CHUL) and has practiced CBT among cancer patients and supervised psychology interns in psycho-oncology for 20 years.

Jennifer Hains, D.Ps. is a psychologist specialized in psycho-oncology. She worked at the breast cancer clinic of the CHU de Québec-Université Laval (Hôpital du St-Sacrement) and now works at L'Hotel-Dieu-de-Quebec part of the CHU de Québec-Université Laval with patients who have different types of cancers. She has provided psychological services to cancer patients using CBT for 5 years.

Part I

Psychotherapy Group on Fear of Cancer Recurrence: Therapist's Manual

Session No. 1

Structure of Session No. 1

Section title	Learning objectives	Page
Introduction	• Introduce the facilitators and identify the creators of the program. • Describe the goals, methods, and themes covered in the program and session no. 1. • Warn participants that the content of the sessions might challenge some of their beliefs about how best to cope with cancer.	4
Information on fear of cancer recurrence	• Define and explain fear of cancer recurrence and its correlates. • Present and illustrate the vicious circle of fear of cancer recurrence and how the program can help break it.	10
Beliefs about the influence of psychological factors on cancer	• Demystify certain beliefs about the influence of psychological factors on cancer (stress = cancer; positive thinking = cure). • Present the multifactorial model of cancer.	14
The cognitive model of emotions	• Explain how thoughts influence emotions. • Present the vicious circle of positive thinking (the tyranny of positive thinking). • Explain the possible negative effects of positive thinking and unrealistic optimism on adjustment to cancer.	30

Supplementary Information: The online version contains supplementary material available at [https://doi.org/10.1007/978-3-031-07187-4_1].

© The Author(s), under exclusive license to Springer Nature Switzerland AG 2022
J. Savard et al., *Treating Fear of Cancer Recurrence with Group Cognitive-Behavioural Therapy: A Step-by-Step Guide*,
https://doi.org/10.1007/978-3-031-07187-4_1

Section title	Learning objectives	Page
The benefits of realistic thinking	• Present the glasses analogy to illustrate negative thoughts (dark glasses) and positive thoughts (rose-coloured glasses). • Present realistic thinking (clear glasses) as an alternative and explain its benefits (to be illustrated using clinical vignettes).	44
Cognitive-behavioural therapy	• Explain what cognitive-behavioural therapy is along with its demonstrated effectiveness.	57
Recognizing negative thoughts	• Present the characteristics of negative thoughts and why it is important to learn to identify them. • Suggest a thought identification exercise to do at home.	59
End of session discussion	• Ask participants what they took away from the session. • Answer questions and summarize key concepts as needed.	63

1.1 Introduction

1.1.1 Slide #1: Fear of Cancer Recurrence

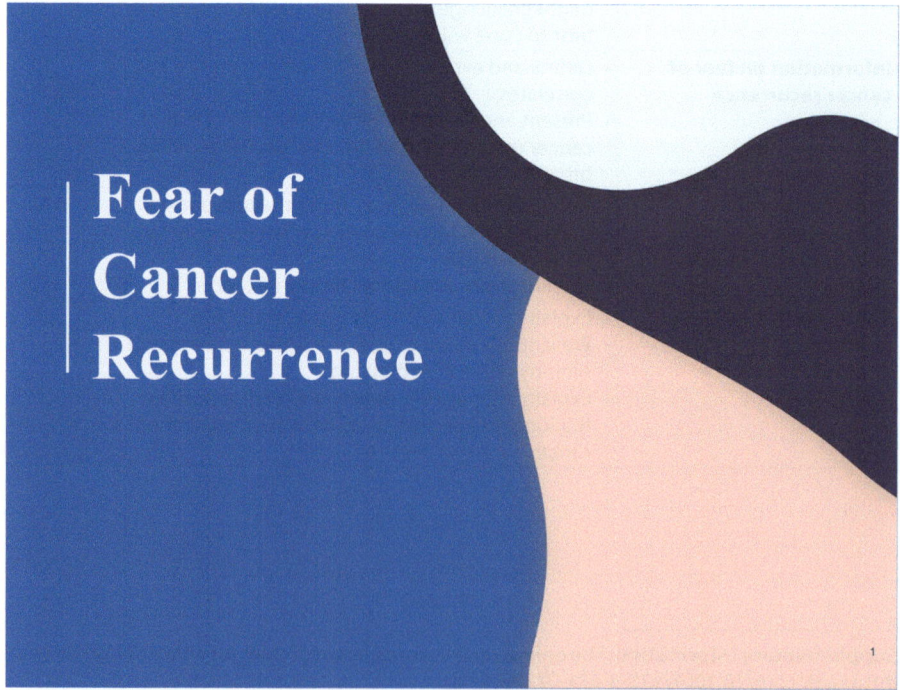

First of all, welcome the group participants and introduce yourself.

1.1 Introduction

1.1.2 Slide #2: Psychotherapy Group on Fear of Cancer Recurrence

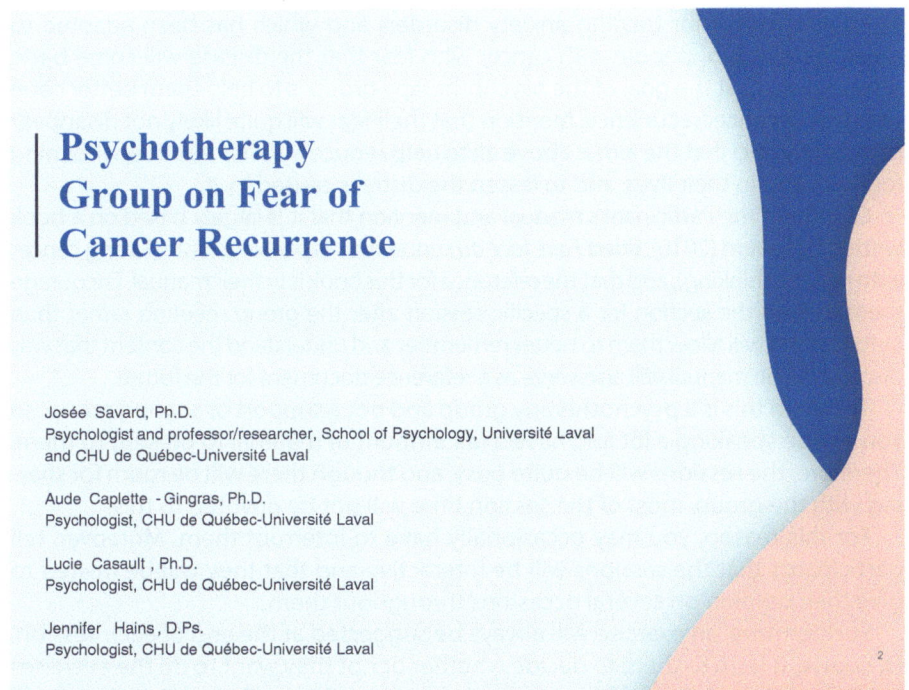

Explain that the psychotherapy group on fear of recurrence was created by Aude Caplette-Gingras, PhD, Lucie Casault, PhD, and Jennifer Hains, PhD, psychologists specialized in oncology at the CHU de Québec-Université Laval, as well as by Josée Savard, PhD, psychologist and professor/researcher at the School of Psychology of Université Laval and at the CHU de Québec-Université Laval. This program was developed because the prevalence of fear of cancer recurrence is high and studies show that it is among the least well-met needs of patients.

Afterwards, explain that the group format was favoured because it allows reaching many people at the same time. Group interventions also allow participants to see that they are not the only ones to have these types of experiences or concerns, which gives them the opportunity to see how other people cope with cancer. Each session will last approximately 90–120 min, and there will be a break taken halfway.

Inform the participants that the psychotherapy group is not only based on clinical experience but also scientific evidence. The proposed interventions are based on an intervention model, cognitive-behavioural therapy, which has been recognized as effective for treating anxiety disorders and which has been adapted to meet the needs of people with cancer who fear that the disease will come back. Also, explain that the goal of the psychotherapy group is to help them better cope with fear of cancer recurrence. Mention that their fear will quite likely not disappear completely and that the aim is above all to help reduce it so it is less overwhelming for them and in their lives, and to lessen the distress caused by it.

Give them the Participant's manual and mention that it is largely based on a book written by Savard (2010), titled *Faire face au cancer avec la pensée réaliste* (Facing cancer with realistic thinking), and that the reference for this book is in their manual. Encourage them to read the section for a specific session after the group meeting rather than before as this will allow them to better remember and understand the content that was discussed. The manual will also serve as a reference document for the future.

Tell them this is a psychotherapy group and not a support or sharing group, so you will be speaking a lot and have a fair amount of material to present to them. Therefore, the sessions will be quite busy, and though there will be room for sharing with the group, most of the session time will not be devoted to this.

For this reason, you may occasionally have to interrupt them. Moreover, tell participants that the sessions will be interactive and that they will be invited to give their opinion on several occasions throughout them.

Furthermore, an exercise will always be suggested at the end of each session. Of course, it is up to them to decide whether or not they want to do the exercises but be sure to point out that by doing them, they truly maximize their chances of reaping the benefits of the program. Their commitment to therapy is a factor of success. Learning new strategies for dealing with anxiety is a bit like learning how to ride a bike: We may understand all the steps involved in keeping our balance and moving forward, but it is only when we try it that we can determine whether or not we can do it, and only with practice can we become more skilful.

Finally, tell them the program has been offered since 2012, and positive results have been observed (Savard et al., 2018).

Before starting the session, invite the participants to briefly introduce themselves and mention where they are in their care trajectory if they are comfortable doing so. Take this opportunity to specify that all participants should keep the content of the group discussions confidential.

1.1 Introduction

1.1.3   Slide #3: Warning

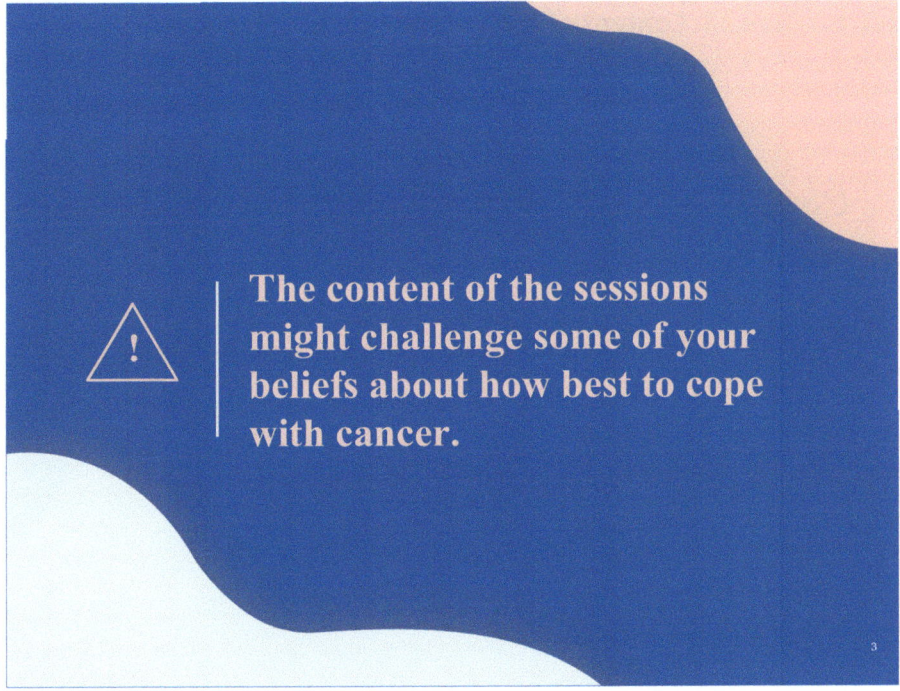

The content of the sessions might challenge some of your beliefs about how best to cope with cancer.

At this time, the facilitator is encouraged to mention the following to the participants:

> **Facilitator:** Before we dive into the topic of our session, we would like to begin with a little warning. Our experience has shown us that some people can be somewhat shaken by the fact that some of the things we say during the sessions are quite different from what is often conveyed about cancer in society. The goal here is to invite you to open your mind to the different perspectives that we offer. After all, if you are here, it is probably because the way you are dealing with your fear of recurrence is not 100% effective. Therefore, we would like to propose another way of going about it, another way of seeing things. This warning is also meant to inform you that your fear of recurrence may seem worse in the following week(s). Know that this is completely normal because our natural reflex to reduce this fear is often to try to avoid thinking or talking about it, while we will instead be talking about it here for two hours a week over four weeks. So, you will probably think about it more. This is a phenomenon that usually fades over time. You might even hesitate to come back for the next session and consider dropping out of the group due to this increase in anxiety. Again, this is a normal reaction. However, we encourage you to continue so you can get to try new strategies to help you better deal with your fear of recurrence. However, if this becomes too difficult for you, it would be important to let us know.

1.2 Content of the Sessions

1.2.1 Slide #4: Content of the Sessions

Content of the Sessions

- Understanding the vicious circle of fear of cancer recurrence (FCR)
- Does thought influence cancer?
- Better managing emotions with realistic optimism
- Learning to tolerate uncertainty
- Demystifying beliefs about the usefulness of worrying
- Facing fears
- What if a recurrence occurs?
- Redefining life goals

Present to participants the general topics that will be covered over the four sessions:

- **Understanding the vicious circle of fear of cancer recurrence**
- **Does thought influence cancer?**
- **Better managing emotions with realistic optimism**
- **Learning to tolerate uncertainty**
- **Demystifying beliefs about the usefulness of worrying**
- **Facing fears**
- **What if a recurrence occurs?**
- **Redefining life goals**

1.2 Content of the Sessions

Possible question from participants:

> **Participant:** Does this intervention work for people for whom the likelihood of a recurrence is high?

> **Facilitator:** That is a good question! Studies show that the likelihood or the real risk of recurrence has little influence on fear intensity. Some people have a 5% risk of recurrence and experience very intense fear, while others have a 50% risk or more, and they tolerate this fact very well. Either way, all the strategies we will propose throughout this program are applicable and can be effective.

1.2.2 Slide #5: Session No. 1

Session No.1

Information on fear of cancer recurrence

The influence of psychological factors
    Does stress cause cancer?
    Can the power of thought cure cancer?

The benefits of realistic thinking
    The tyranny of positive thinking
    Realistic thinking and cancer

Cognitive - behavioural therapy

 Identification of negative thoughts exercise

Next, present the specific plan of the session:

- **Information on fear of cancer recurrence**
- **The influence of psychological factors**
    - Does stress cause cancer?
    - Can the power of thought cure cancer?
- **The benefits of realistic thinking**
    - The tyranny of positive thinking
    - Realistic thinking and cancer
- **Cognitive-behavioural therapy**
- **Identification of negative thoughts exercise**

1.3 Information on Fear of Cancer Recurrence

Section objectives:

- **Define fear of recurrence.**
- **Understand the difference between normal and pathological fear of recurrence.**
- **Present the characteristics of pathological fear of recurrence:**
    - Constant
    - Overwhelming (altered functioning)
    - Intense (notable distress)
    - Lasts over time
- **Identify the factors associated with the development of fear of recurrence:**
    - Female sex
    - Young age
    - Many side effects and physical symptoms
    - Anxious temperament
- **Present the vicious circle of fear of recurrence:**
    - Internal/external cues, knowledge about cancer
    - Interpretation
    - Coping strategies that are ineffective over the long term (avoidance, seeking reassurance and control)
    - Intolerance of uncertainty

1.3 Information on Fear of Cancer Recurrence

1.3.1 Slide #6: Fear of Cancer Recurrence

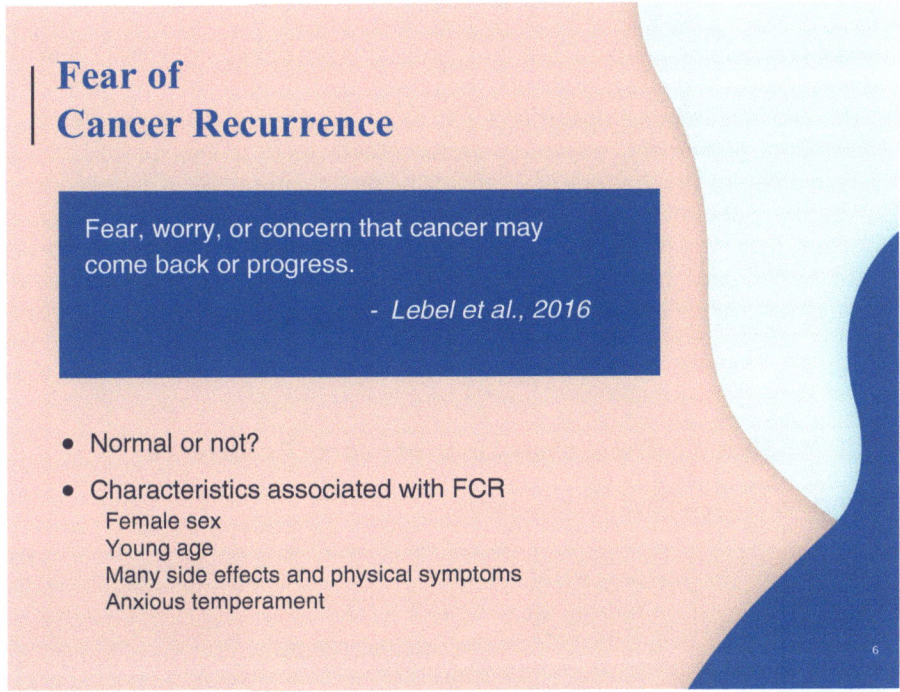

Explain the following about fear of recurrence:

Facilitator: In 2016, a group of international experts ruled that fear of cancer recurrence is: "fear, worry, or concern that cancer may come back or progress" (Lebel et al., 2016). Fear of recurrence affects just about everyone who has been treated for cancer; therefore, it can be a normal reaction. Fear of recurrence that is considered "normal" is generally mild, easy to control, and might increase as medical follow-ups approach, but quickly decrease after receiving normal test results. The fear is considered more problematic (or "pathological") when it is associated with a lot of distress, suffering, or reduced functioning in different areas of the person's life, whether at work or in their personal life, or when it lasts over time, that is, when it remains intense and overwhelming for months or even years. In such cases, an intervention is necessary.

Next, identify some characteristics that available studies have shown to be associated with fear of recurrence.

> **Facilitator:** Some people are at greater risk of developing problematic fear of recurrence. This is especially the case for women, younger patients, people who experience more side effects and physical symptoms, and people of anxious temperament. Indeed, if a person already tends to experience anxiety in different areas of their life, they will be particularly at risk of experiencing anxiety about cancer as well. However, these factors, called predisposing factors, may help increase the likelihood of experiencing fear of recurrence but are not enough to trigger it. It is really once a vicious circle has set in that fear of recurrence will persist and perhaps even intensify over time.

1.3.2 Slide #7: The Vicious Circle of Fear of Recurrence

The vicious circle of fear of recurrence

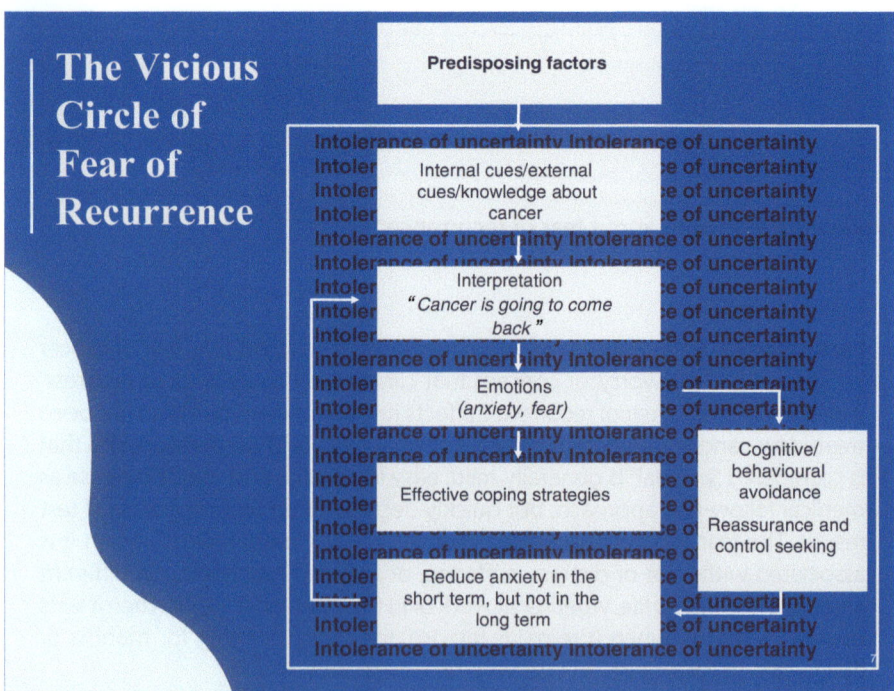

Present the vicious circle of fear of recurrence as follows:

Facilitator: In general, fear of recurrence will arise in reaction to certain cues. The cues can be internal, such as a physical symptom (e.g. pain) or certain memories. For example, you have a headache and are worried because you have had cancer before, and you think it might have come back. Symptoms that are quite likely to cause fear of recurrence are often the same ones that led to the initial diagnosis. Further, cues can also be external. For example, you see a television report on cancer and feel like changing the channel because the topic arouses fear in you. Because cancer is not a rare disease and we often hear about it, you are regularly exposed to this kind of cue. The fear can also be fuelled by knowledge, or a lack of knowledge, about cancer in general and about the specific type of cancer you had. For example, when a person does not know whether a symptom might be a sign of recurrence, they are more likely to worry about it.

Facilitator: These different cues tend to lead to catastrophic interpretations, such as concluding that cancer will come back or that it already has come back. This thought or interpretation will in turn generate negative emotions such as anxiety, fear, guilt, helplessness, sadness, or anger. Human beings often react to these unpleasant emotions by trying to make them disappear as quickly as possible, for example, by practicing avoidance. There are different forms of avoidance, including cognitive avoidance and behavioural avoidance. Cognitive avoidance involves trying to drive away thoughts that make you uncomfortable or that cause you distress, while behavioural avoidance involves trying to avoid situations that remind you of the disease. For example, changing the channel when there is a television report on cancer or not going to the same supermarket as usual because you do not want to cross paths with a person who might ask you about your disease. Moreover, to reduce anxiety or distress, some people will seek reassurance. For example, calling their nurse to ask if a symptom that they have is normal, or asking a friend or a partner if they think everything is okay. Also, because cancer can make people feel that they lost a certain degree of control over their life, they may try to regain some control by making drastic lifestyle changes (e.g. stop drinking alcohol). Unfortunately, these strategies are only effective in reducing anxiety in the short term. Indeed, when we change the television channel, when we are reassured by others, or when we manage to stop drinking alcohol, our anxiety instantly decreases. However, the fear will come back just as strong when we face external or internal cues again, which will then, once again, trigger the vicious circle of fear of recurrence. Therefore, this program aims to help you adopt strategies that will be more effective in the long term, such as changing your way of interpreting things, practising less avoidance, and seeking less reassurance and control in an attempt to block the vicious circle of fear of recurrence. In this regard, we will propose different strategies throughout the sessions.

> **Facilitator:** Finally, as you can see, intolerance of uncertainty, or what is often called "allergy to uncertainty," is shown in the background. It is often observed in anxious patients; they have a much lower tolerance of uncertainty. When they do not know what the future holds, they become uncomfortable and anxious. Not knowing for sure whether cancer will come back is often intolerable for these people. A person's baseline level of tolerance of uncertainty will considerably influence the different components of the circle. We will go over each of these concepts over the next sessions.

At this point, ask participants if they have any questions or comments.

1.4 Beliefs About the Influence of Psychological Factors on Cancer

Section objectives:

- **Demystify some popular beliefs about the causes of cancer.**
- **Explain the importance of relying on results obtained in scientific literature rather than on ideas conveyed in pop psychology books. Scientific research:**
    - Uses large and diversified samples
    - Is objective
    - Is replicable

1.4 Beliefs About the Influence of Psychological Factors on Cancer

1.4.1   Slide #8: The Vicious Circle of Fear of Recurrence

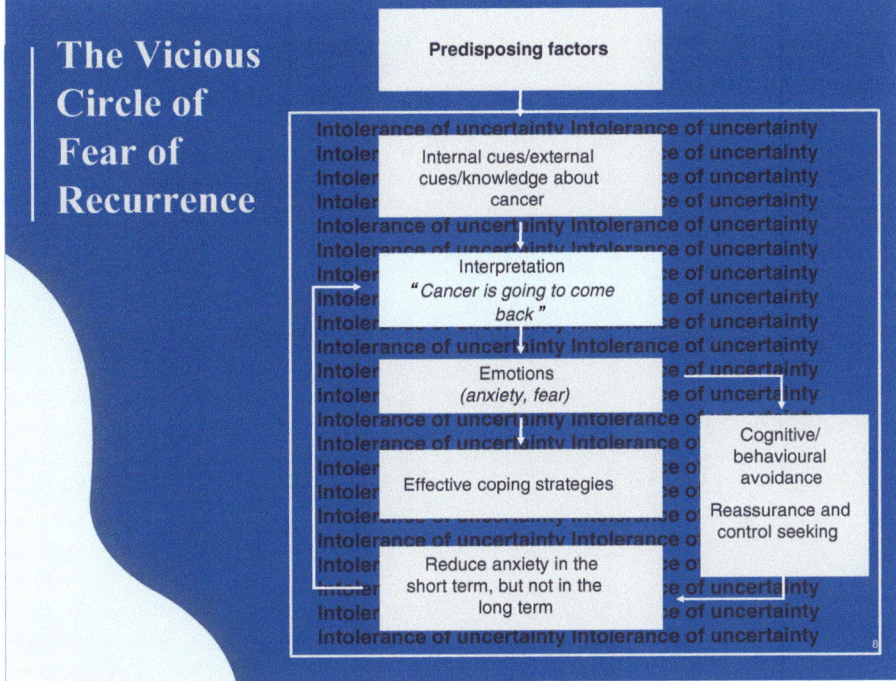

Tell participants the following:

Facilitator: Although it is possible to intervene on several other components of the model, we will focus on the "Interpretation" box, that is, the one concerning thoughts, for the rest of the session.

1.4.2 Slide #9: The Power of Thought

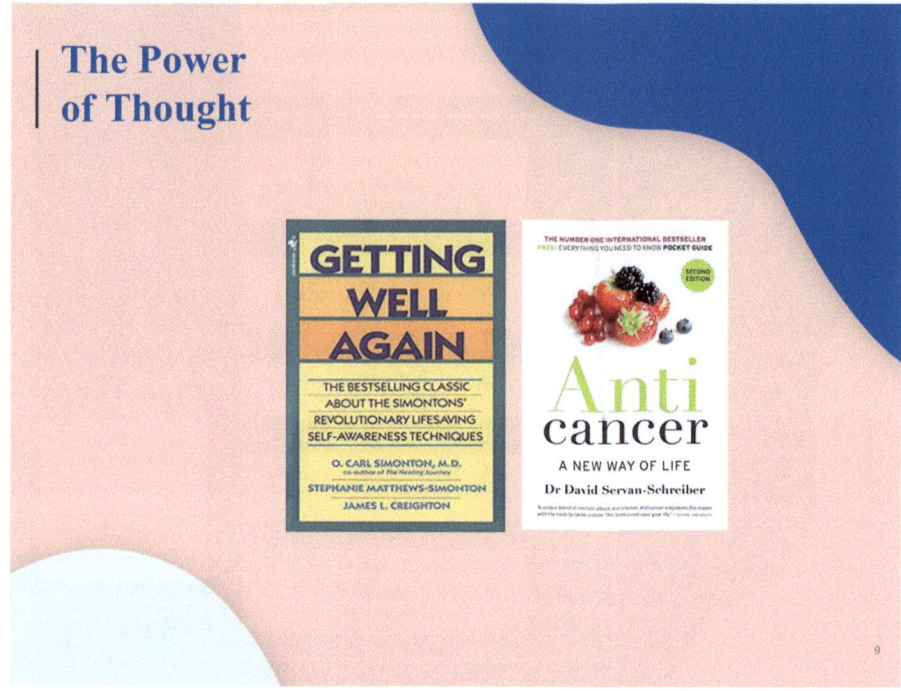

Facilitator: Much has been written about the role of thoughts in coping with cancer and even on their influence on the likelihood of being cured. You have probably all seen or read these types of publications at the library or at the bookstore, namely, pop psychology books that often highlight two ideas.

1.4.3 Slide #10: Influence of Psychological Factors on Cancer

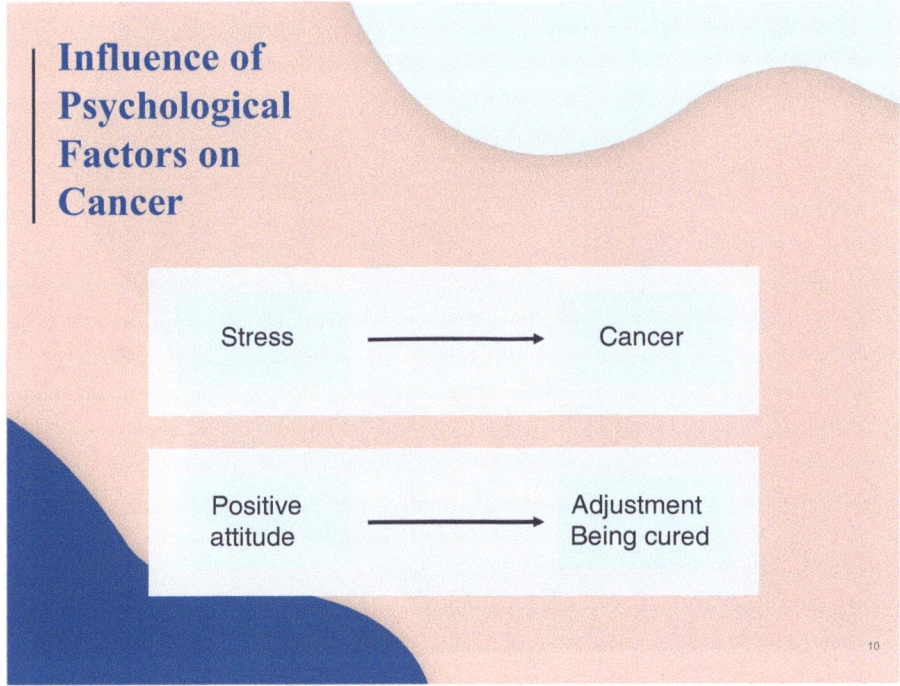

Facilitator: The first idea is that stress and other psychological factors, such as depression, loneliness, or having experienced a traumatic event, increase the risk of cancer. The second idea is that a person's mental attitude plays a decisive role in the progression of cancer and influences the chances of being cured. More specifically, it is advocated that having a positive attitude will increase one's chances not only of adjusting better to cancer but also of being cured.

1.4.4 Slide #11: Popular Beliefs

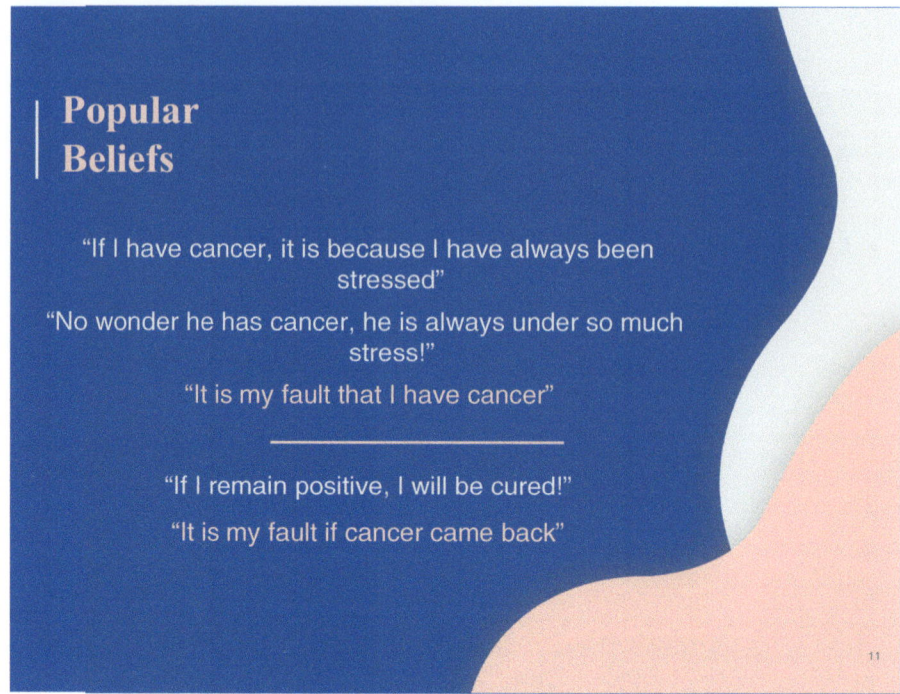

Facilitator: These beliefs are also quite widespread in the population. Concerning the first belief, we may have heard things such as: "If I have cancer, it is because I have always been stressed" or "No wonder he has cancer, he is always under so much stress." However, there is a negative counterpart to this belief, which is the tendency to feel guilty about having cancer because we believe it is due to our inability to deal with stress. Further, there is also a negative counterpart to the second belief. On the one hand, we may feel that it gives us hope: if we manage to remain positive, we will be cured of cancer. On the other hand, if cancer comes back, or if we are afraid that it will, we might think that it is or would be our fault because we do not have the right mental attitude. It is common in clinical practice to see people who seek psychological counselling because their cancer came back, and they feel guilty about it.

1.4.5 Slide #12: Clinical Cases vs. Scientific Research

Clinical Cases vs. Scientific Research

Clinical cases
- Few, selected cases, that confirm our theory
- What about the others?

Scientific research
- Large groups of people with various characteristics
- The only way to verify whether an idea or a theory is true

Facilitator: Today, we will find out whether these beliefs are based on facts. If you have read pop psychology books such as those presented earlier, you already know that the authors of these books often discuss specific cases. A typical example is that of a person who had a poor prognosis, so who was very unlikely to be cured of their cancer, yet they still managed to recover with the power of their mind. Conversely, they could also describe the case of a person with a negative attitude for whom a recurrence was unlikely, but whose disease nevertheless progressed quite quickly. For people with cancer, these examples are often quite convincing, because they are relatable to them. However, because these authors wish to convince you that their theory is true (and they are convinced of this themselves), they will necessarily describe clinical cases that confirm their theory. They will not write about the hundreds or thousands of other cases they have seen that did not support their theory. Therefore, the only way to verify whether an idea or theory is true is through scientific research. We will not tell you about all the studies that have been published as this would be too tedious and time-consuming, but we will describe a few studies that have focused on these two hypotheses, that is, whether stress causes cancer and whether positive thinking increases the chances of curing cancer. Scientific research has the advantage of focusing on large groups of people rather than on just a few cases without considering what happens to the others. Therefore, it is possible to verify whether it is true, for example, that people who have experienced more stressful events have a higher chance of developing cancer.

1.5 Stress = Cancer?

Section objectives:

- **Present the factors involved or suspected of being involved in the etiology of cancer with the multifactorial model of cancer.**
- **Explain that scientific studies do not currently conclude that stress or other psychological factors can cause cancer.**
- **Emphasize that there is still much to be discovered about the causes of cancer.**
- **Point out that just because the medical cause of a disease is unknown or unclear does not mean it is necessarily psychological (e.g. stomach ulcers).**

1.5 Stress = Cancer?

1.5.1 Slide #13: Stress → Cancer?

| Stress → Cancer ?

In the vast majority of cases, no link between stress and cancer has been demonstrated

STRESS

- Role of lifestyle habits
  stress → less healthy habits → cancer
- Who does not experience stress?
- Does it explain cancer in children?
- Associated with ↓ of immune system, but its impact remains unknown on cancer
- According to cancer organizations, stress is not identified as a known/possible risk factor
- The absence of a known biological cause does not mean that it is psychological (*stomach ulcers*)

Present the following information concerning the influence of thoughts on cancer. Mention that the idea according to which stress or other psychological factors can cause cancer is not new. This question has been studied since the 1960s and has been the focus of several dozens and even hundreds of studies. By examining the literature, it is certainly possible to identify some studies that have shown that people who are highly stressed are also more vulnerable to cancer. However, it is essential to specify to participants that when all the literature is considered, that is, all the studies that were carried out on this subject, it is clear that in the vast majority of cases, no link between stress (or other psychological factors) and cancer has been demonstrated (Coyne et al., 2010). Therefore, since it is the exception rather than the rule that has shown a link, one must conclude that the literature does not provide strong support for this hypothesis.

Also, explain that studies that have shown a link rarely took into account the fact that people whose living conditions are more stressful also tend to have less healthy lifestyle habits. For example, we can easily imagine that a person living in a context of great poverty will have less healthy eating habits, exercise less, and tend to smoke, and such habits are factors that increase the risk of cancer. Therefore, it is not so much stress per se, but rather the lifestyle habits associated with stress that increase the risk of cancer. To support this point, you can describe the results of a Danish population study that showed a slight increase in cancer risk in people who had survived deportation to a German concentration camp during the Second World War, and who had thus been subjected to extreme stress (Olsen et al., 2015). However, this effect was found only for cancers related to smoking or alcohol use, such as those of the lung or of the head and neck. Consequently, this shows that stress as such is not what causes cancer.

Next, ask who among the participants has not experienced stress over the last week. Normally, nobody should raise their hand. Tell them that stress has always been a part of life. Even the "prehistoric man" experienced stress, albeit of a different nature (e.g. finding food, ensuring his survival and safety, etc.). Tell them that 100% of people experience stress, and if it were truly associated with cancer, it would not be close to one in two people who would develop cancer in their lifetime, but 100%. You could also mention the example of young children with cancer. It is difficult to believe that stress could have played a major role in the development of their disease.

Next, mention the following to participants:

> **Facilitator:** Often, in pop psychology books, it is mentioned that research has shown that stress weakens the immune system, which in turn increases the risk of cancer. A part of this assertion is true. Indeed, it is true that scientific literature has shown that stress is associated with alterations of the immune system and with a higher risk of developing certain infections (e.g. the common cold). Studies conducted among university students have shown that during exam weeks, so when stress is present, they are much more likely to develop a cold or the flu than at the start of the semester. Stress is also a known risk factor for cardiovascular disease, an effect that could be due to changes in the immune system (inflammation). But what has not yet been demonstrated is whether changes in the immune system associated with stress, depression or other psychological factors are of a nature, an intensity, and a duration that are significant enough to have an impact on a disease as complex as cancer. We will go over this point later on in the session.

Possible question from participants:

> **Participant:** Is cancer really linked to the immune system?

> **Facilitator:** The idea that the immune system is involved in all types of cancer is controversial. We know that it is involved in the development of cancers of a viral nature, such as cervical cancer, which is associated with the human papillomavirus (HPV). Furthermore, immunotherapy for some types of cancer, the effectiveness of which is currently being studied, appears to produce good results, which suggests that the immune system could be involved in curing cancer. In short, the immune system's role in the etiology or progression of cancer is not yet fully understood.

1.5 Stress = Cancer?

At this point, ask participants if they have ever asked their oncologist why they developed cancer and what answer they were given. Doctors often respond that it is impossible for them to know, which is an answer that can be quite baffling for patients. Explain that when no specific biological cause can be identified, people tend to try to find a psychological cause to their disease, which is a completely normal reaction. However, the absence of a known biological cause of their disease does not necessarily mean that the cause is psychological. Give the example of stomach ulcers: for decades, people thought they were due to stress until it was discovered that most of them were caused by a form of bacteria (*Helicobacter pylori*) that can be treated effectively with antibiotics. Tell them that despite many scientific breakthroughs, there is still much that has yet to be discovered about cancer, and in the meantime, it is essential to avoid concluding that it is caused by psychological factors.

At this point, and before presenting the Multifactorial Model of Cancer figure, ask participants what they know about risk factors for cancer. Encourage them to give several examples.

Here are various examples of answers that participants could give, as well as feedback suggestions that facilitators could use in response to these answers:

- **Tobacco use:** Tell participants that this is indeed a major risk factor for lung cancer, but it is also associated with other cancers such as cervical and head and neck cancer.
- **Genetics:** Tell them that 5% to 10% of cancers are of genetic origin, namely, certain breast and ovarian cancers.
- **Hormones:** Tell them that it is true that the number of years of exposure to oestrogen and progesterone can increase the risk of developing breast or ovarian cancer. For example, having an early first period and late menopause, or having used hormone replacement therapy during menopause, increases the risk of having one of these cancers.
- **Environment:** Explain that this element has been studied, but there is little firm evidence available about it. It is indeed difficult to identify precise environmental factors that play a specific role in the development of cancer because we are exposed daily to electromagnetic fields, various chemicals, etc. However, asbestos is an exception because it clearly increases the risk of several cancers, especially lung cancer.
- **Diet:** Tell them that this factor is indeed often discussed, especially in the media. Some even speak of anticancer diets. However, we must remain cautious so as to avoid making overly categorical judgments about the role of nutrition. Explain that based on the available and often conflicting data, it is difficult to determine which foods should be avoided and which ones should

be consumed in order to avoid developing cancer. Just because a certain substance (e.g. turmeric) has shown anticancer properties in test tubes does not mean that the same goes for the human body. Therefore, we do not know exactly how much turmeric should be consumed to obtain a real beneficial effect. Moreover, both laboratory and nutrition studies fail to take into account the fact that humans do not eat only one type of food, which means that interaction effects are possible between all the foods that we consume (e.g. if on one hand I eat X g of turmeric, but on the other hand I have X alcoholic drinks or I eat a lot of red meat, does the effect cancel out?). Also, tell them that nutritional organizations still concludes that to stay healthy, it is best to have a varied and balanced diet in order to get as many nutrients as possible.

- **Viruses:** Tell them that some viruses can indeed increase the risk of cancer, such as HPV for cervical cancer or HIV for Kaposi sarcoma.
- **Lack of physical exercise:** Tell them that this is a factor on which we are beginning to gather convincing evidence. But again, it remains difficult to accurately determine the quantity, frequency, and type of exercise that can help prevent cancer.

1.5.2 Slide #14: Multifactorial Model of Cancer

Multifactorial model of cancer

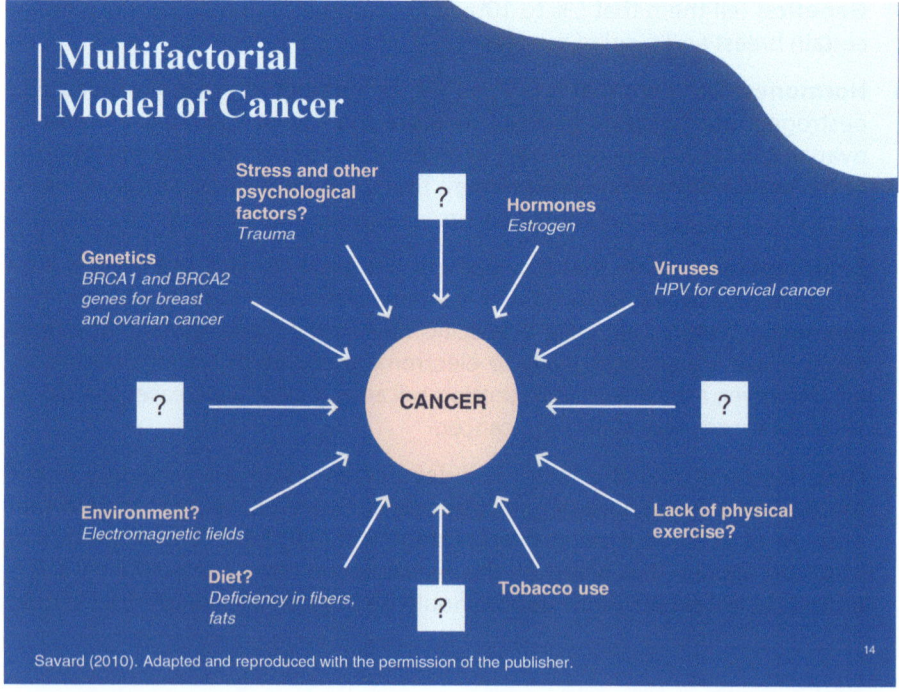

Savard (2010). Adapted and reproduced with the permission of the publisher.

Present the Multifactorial Model of Cancer and briefly go over the other risk factors illustrated in the figure that were not identified by participants.

> **Facilitator:** The takeaway of this figure is not so much its specific elements but rather the idea that cancer is a multifactorial disease. In other words, it is influenced by a whole set of factors that vary from one type of cancer to another (there are over 200 types of cancer), and from one person to another. For example, if we consider the cases of two women with breast cancer, the disease may mostly be due to genetic factors for one, and for the other, it may be due to hormonal factors or lifestyle habits. In short, we can compare cancer to a recipe that contains several ingredients that vary in nature and quantity from one to another. There is no single recipe for developing cancer, just as there is no single recipe for cake.

> **Facilitator:** Something else to remember is that all the question marks indicate that there is still much that we do not yet know about the causes of cancer. Despite everything that we said previously, we still included stress and other psychological factors in the model and added a question mark next to them. The bottom line is if these factors do influence cancer, it would be through the effect of many other known or even unknown factors that are much more influential. Therefore, the association is much more complex than stress = cancer.

Are there any questions or comments about this?

1.6 Positive Thoughts = Cure?

Section objectives:

- **Explain that studies show that a person's mental attitude does not appear to have a decisive role on the initial development of cancer or its progression.**
- **Emphasize that scientific literature shows that firmly believing that stress causes cancer or that positive thinking can cure cancer are associated with more psychological distress and fear of recurrence.**
- **Help participants understand that fear of recurrence and psychological distress are likely to affect their quality of life, and although psychotherapy will not help cure their cancer, it can still help them cope better with the disease.**

1.6.1 Slide #15: Mental Attitude and Cancer Survival – Study 1

Mental Attitude and Cancer Survival

STUDY 1
- Women with metastatic breast cancer
- 50 patients received psychotherapy vs. 36 did not
- Group psychotherapy: expression of emotions, support between participants
- Intervention improves quality of life, ↓ distress

- Spiegel's group therapy
  Survival:
     With therapy: 36.6 months
     Without therapy: 18.9 months

Present the study of American psychiatrist David Spiegel, published in 1989. Explain that the study focused on women with metastatic breast cancer (i.e. advanced breast cancer with no chance of being cured). About half of the women attended group psychotherapy once a week for a year, and the other half did not. At the end of the study, the authors found, as expected, that participation in the psychotherapy group reduced psychological distress, namely, depressive and anxiety symptoms. An even more astonishing observation was that women who received the psychological intervention had lived twice as long as those who did not receive it, that is, on average 37 months compared to 19. From that point on, the media began spreading the message that psychotherapy could cure cancer and that mental attitude could help beat the disease.

At this point, issue the following warning:

Facilitator: However, researchers have generally received these results with great caution because, in research, a phenomenon must be observed in more than one study before we can conclude that it is real. Indeed, a result must be observed and replicated in multiple studies, carried out by several research teams (a process called "replication"). Hence, researchers have pointed out the importance of replicating these results in other studies.

1.6.2 Slide #16: Mental Attitude and Cancer Survival – Study 2

Mental Attitude and Cancer Survival

STUDY 1	STUDY 2
• Women with metastatic breast cancer	• Women with metastatic breast cancer
• 50 patients received psychotherapy vs. 36 did not	• **158 patients received psychotherapy vs. 77 did not**
• Group psychotherapy: expression of emotions, support between participants	• Group psychotherapy: expression of emotions, support between participants
• Intervention improves quality of life, ↓ distress	• Intervention improves quality of life, ↓ distress: especially in women with high levels of distress

• Spiegel's group therapy
 	
Survival:
  With therapy: 36.6 months
  Without therapy: 18.9 months
	• Spiegel's group therapy
	
	Survival:
	  With therapy: 17.9 months
	  Without therapy: 17.6 months

Facilitator: Many replication studies have been carried out, including one by Canadian researcher Pamela Goodwin, who essentially conducted the same study as Spiegel, but with a larger number of participants (Goodwin et al., 2001). In other words, it was a more rigorous study conducted once again with women with metastatic breast cancer. Two-thirds of the women received psychotherapy for one year, and the others did not. An interesting fact about this study is that the therapists who administered the psychological intervention, which was the exact same intervention that was administered in the original study conducted by Spiegel, had been trained by Spiegel himself. The results showed a decrease in psychological distress at the end of the psychotherapy, especially in women who had higher levels of it at the start of the study. Concerning survival, no difference was found between the two groups. Many other replication studies have since been published, but none to this day has managed to replicate the original results obtained by Spiegel.

1.6.3 Slide #17: Why Is It Important to Let Go of These Beliefs?

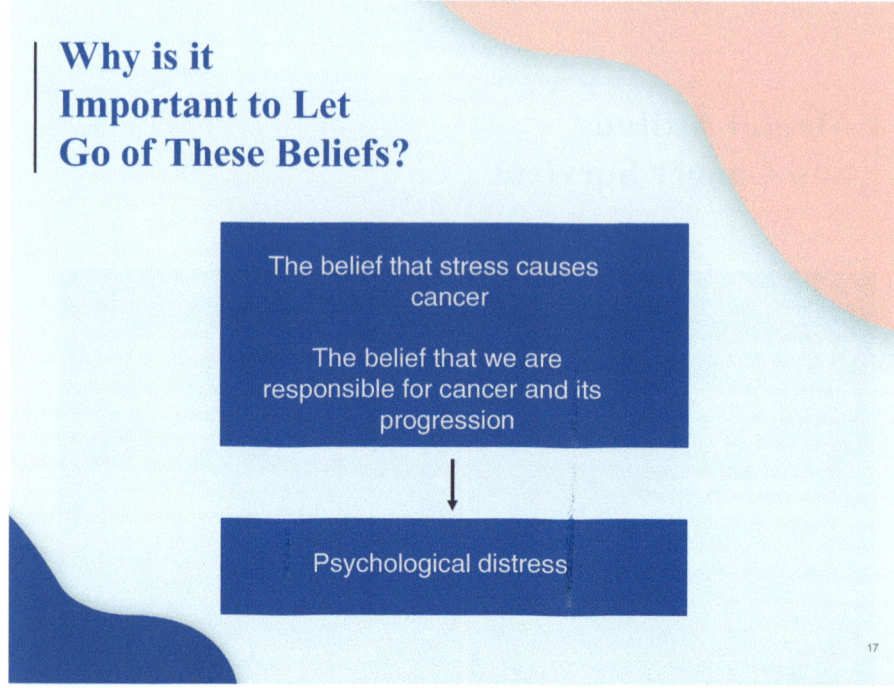

At this point, explain to participants why it is important to let go of the beliefs that stress causes cancer or that mental attitude plays a determining role in its progression. Explain that scientific literature shows that such beliefs are associated with higher psychological distress, so with more depressive and anxiety symptoms, and a higher level of fear of cancer recurrence (Dumalaon-Canaria et al., 2018; Pedersen et al., 2012). However, specify that if they hold these beliefs and are reluctant to let them go completely, it would be wise to at least have some doubts about them. Indeed, giving less credit to these beliefs or adopting a more nuanced view about them may help them experience fewer psychological symptoms, including fear of cancer recurrence. Remind them that they do not need to fully agree with what is said during the sessions but that questioning these beliefs even minimally and seeing them less as certainties can be helpful.

1.6 Positive Thoughts = Cure?   29

1.6.4   Slide #18: Summary

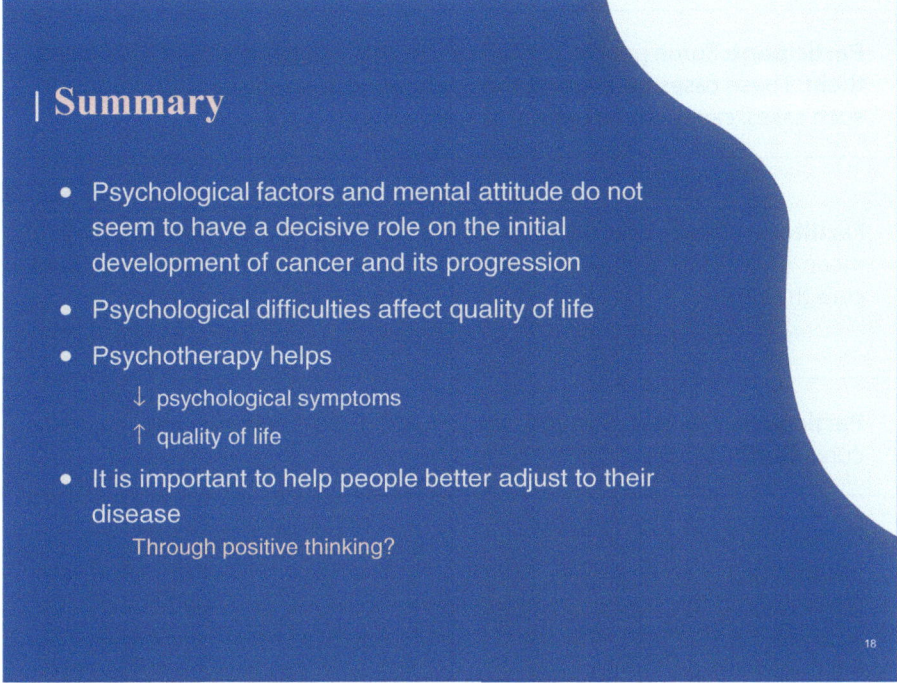

Briefly summarize this section for participants by telling them that psychological factors and mental attitude do not seem to have a decisive role on the initial development of cancer or on its progression. Choose the words you use carefully. It is important to use terms such as "do not seem" because science evolves. Then, tell them that it is nevertheless recognized that psychological difficulties, such as fear of recurrence, affect quality of life and that psychotherapy helps reduce psychological distress and improve quality of life. Hence, the psychotherapy they are currently receiving will not cure them, but it should help them better adjust to their disease. Finish by saying that in the following minutes, the question of whether positive thinking is an effective strategy for coping with cancer will be discussed.

At this point, ask participants if they have any questions or comments.

Possible question from participants:

> **Participant:** Some people survive cancer that ordinarily would have killed them. These cases go beyond the limits of both science and the body. In such cases, can it not be helpful to have a fighting attitude?

> **Facilitator:** The answer depends on the meaning of your question: do you mean could it help a person get through the situation or could it help cure them?

> **Participant:** To get through the situation but perhaps also to help cure them?

> **Facilitator:** For some people, having a fighting spirit helps them cope with the disease. If this is your case and this works for you, you need not change anything: we stick with what works for us. However, as we will see later, believing that it is important to maintain a fighting spirit can have harmful effects. Concerning the connections between a fighting spirit and cancer survival, a few studies have been conducted. Although early studies have shown some degree of association, other studies that are both more recent and rigorous have not confirmed these results. Therefore, a fighting spirit does not seem to play a determining role in cancer survival. One possible explanation as to why some people live longer than predicted is that their body, for one reason or another, was able to fight off the specific type of tumour they had. As mentioned previously, just because a phenomenon cannot yet be explained by biology does not mean that it is necessarily psychological. However, the aim here is not to convince you that we possess the absolute truth, but instead to present another way of seeing things and to raise your awareness about the fact that these beliefs can have negative effects.

1.7 The Cognitive Model of Emotions

Section objectives:

- **Emphasize that cancer is a distressing experience that generally leads to negative thoughts and disturbing emotions.**
- **Present the cognitive model of emotions.**
- **Explain that it is not the objective situation as such but rather its interpretation that generates reactions and determines the intensity of the emotions experienced.**

1.7.1 Slide #19: Cancer: A Distressing Experience

Cancer: A Distressing Experience

- Negative thoughts
    I am going to die (cancer = death)
    I am going to suffer and so will my loved ones
    This is unfair!
    It is my fault!

- Disturbing emotions
    Sadness, anxiety, anger, and guilt, etc.

Explain to participants that cancer is a difficult experience that is usually associated with all sorts of negative thoughts. When a person is diagnosed with cancer, a thought that often comes to mind is that they are going to die because cancer is still very much associated with death. You can tell them that this is actually less and less the case because survival rates improve every year. Also, tell them that several other negative thoughts may surface after being diagnosed with cancer, such as: "I am going to suffer and so will my loved ones," "This is unfair," "It is my fault," and so forth. Continue by saying that cancer is also an experience that is likely to generate many negative emotions such as sadness, anxiety, anger, and guilt.

1.7.2 Slide #20: Cognitive Model of Emotions (Beck)

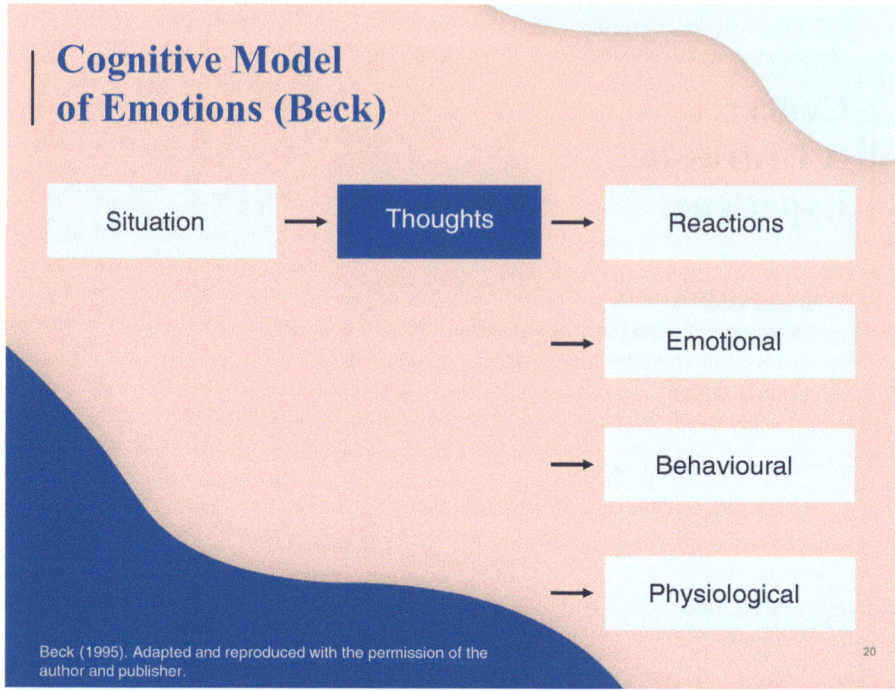

Describe the cognitive model of emotions elaborated by Beck, an eminent American psychiatrist who developed cognitive therapy. First, explain that this model emphasizes the close link between thoughts and emotional, behavioural, and physiological reactions. Tell participants that according to this model, it is not so much a situation per se that generates the reactions or negative emotions that ensue but rather its interpretation, and this is true even for objectively difficult situations such as being diagnosed with cancer. In other words, it is the way we interpret a situation that determines the types of emotions experienced and their intensity.

1.8 The Vicious Circle of the Tyranny of Positive Thinking: The Case of Melissa

Section objectives:

- **Present the vicious circle of positive thinking.**
- **Explain that it is not realistic to have positive thoughts at all times when experiencing a difficult situation such as cancer.**
- **Explain that even if positive thoughts can initially block a negative emotion, this calming effect does not tend to last because such thoughts are hard to believe (reverts to negative thoughts as soon as a doubt arises).**
- **Emphasize the fact that the perpetual mental battle between positive and negative thoughts is exhausting and demands a lot of energy.**

1.8.1 Slides #21–22: The Case of Melissa

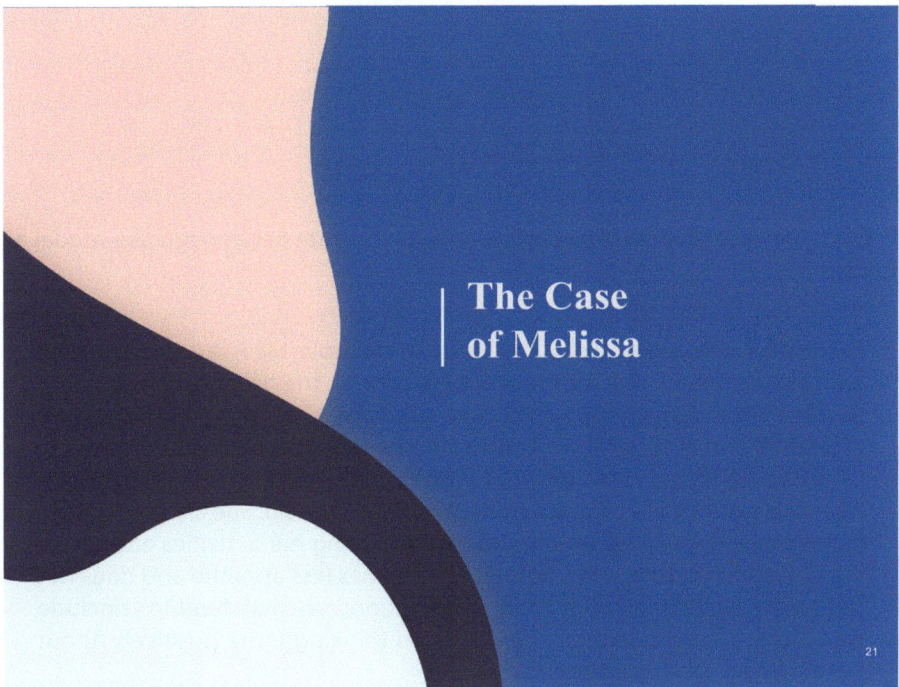

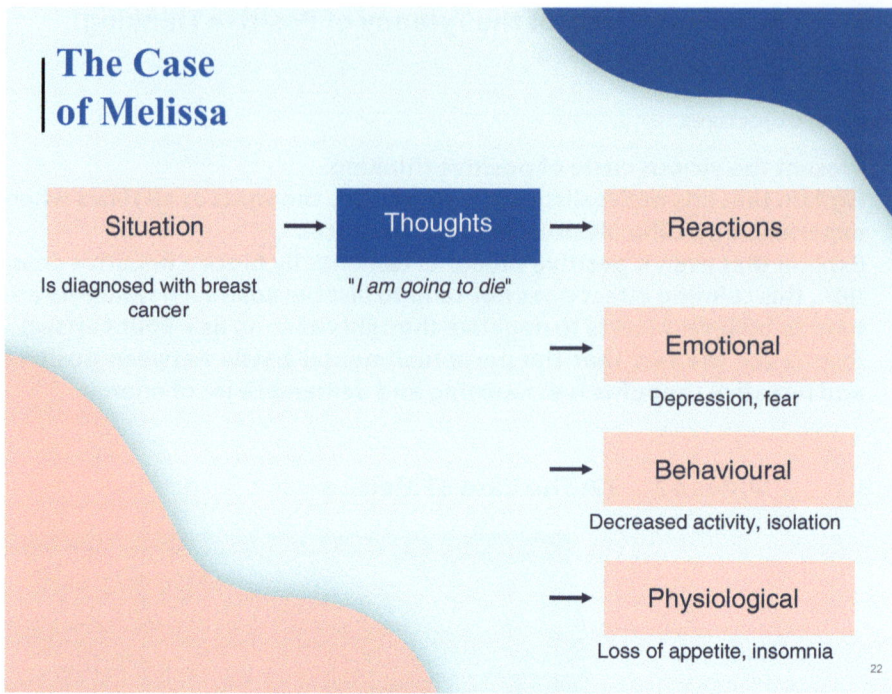

Present the case of Melissa to participants to illustrate Beck's cognitive model as follows:

> **Facilitator:** Let us take Melissa's case as an example. Melissa was diagnosed with breast cancer. Her spontaneous reaction at the time was: "I am going to die." Considering the close link between our interpretations (our thoughts) and reactions, we can easily imagine that because of this very catastrophic thought of hers, her subsequent reactions should be quite negative, right? Melissa is indeed depressed and afraid. She also engages in certain maladaptive behaviours such as reducing her activities and isolating herself from others. Physiologically, she has less appetite and does not sleep very well. Faced with these observations, we may tend to conclude that Melissa would certainly benefit from thinking more positively about her situation. Do you agree?

1.8.2 Slide #23: The Case of Melissa (Continued)

> **The Case of Melissa**
>
> Melissa is currently being treated for breast cancer. She often feels sad and anxious about her prognosis. She has read several books on the power of positive thinking, so she is convinced that her sadness and anxiety will harm her chances of being cured. She feels guilty for not being able to maintain a positive attitude.
>
> "Since I am unable to remain positive, I will surely end up dying from my cancer."
>
> She decides to see a psychologist in an effort to improve her chances of survival.

Facilitator: Before concluding on this, let us continue with the description of Melissa's case. "Melissa is currently being treated for breast cancer. She often feels sad and anxious about her prognosis. She has read several books on the power of positive thinking, so she is convinced that her sadness and anxiety will harm her chances of being cured. She feels guilty for not being able to maintain a positive attitude. She figures that since she is unable to remain positive, she will surely end up dying from her cancer. She decides to see a psychologist in an effort to improve her chances of survival."

1.8.3　Slide #24: The Tyranny of Positive Thinking

The vicious circle of positive thinking

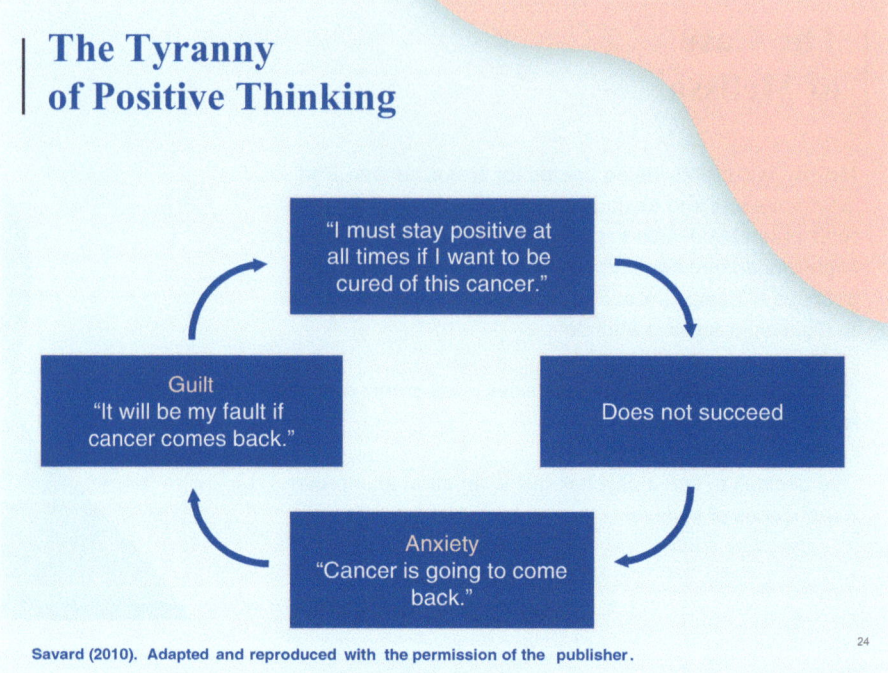

Facilitator: What we see here in Melissa's case is what Jimmie Holland, another American psychiatrist and a pioneer figure in the field of psycho-oncology, called "the tyranny of positive thinking." Savard (2010) went a step further by describing the process through which the tyranny of positive thinking operates. It is a vicious circle that stems from the belief that one must remain positive at all times in order to cure cancer. Like Melissa, many people do not manage to do so. Do you know why?

Participant: Because living with cancer is hard. Cancer treatments are very demanding, and that is why people often do not manage to stay positive. They may feel that they cannot see the end of the tunnel because things keep piling up one after another!

Facilitator: Exactly. It is indeed hard to remain positive when we are experiencing all kinds of symptoms or when we notice that we are not functioning as well as before. And even in the case of a person who is not ill, is it really possible to stay positive all the time?

Participant: No.

Facilitator: So, the vicious circle of positive thinking stems from a very rigid belief about staying positive all the time. Of course, this is an unattainable goal that cannot be achieved by anyone. Believing that their inability to remain positive will have consequences on their health, the person with cancer will feel anxiety and guilt, and may think: "Because I am not being positive enough, cancer will come back" or "If cancer comes back, it will be my fault." Therefore, this belief creates a vicious circle where the more we try to be positive, the less we manage to do so.

1.8.4   Slide #25: Negative Thoughts vs. Positive Thoughts

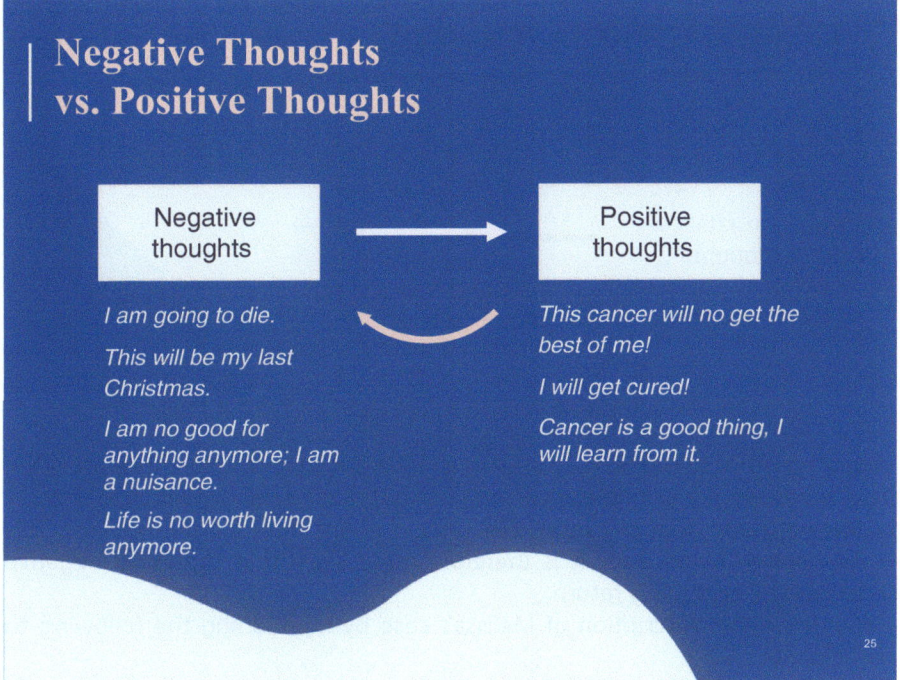

Using Melissa's example, remind participants that cancer can lead to a series of negative thoughts, such as: "I'm going to die," "This will be my last Christmas," "I am no good for anything anymore," "I am a nuisance," or "Life is not worth living anymore." Tell them that typically, one negative thought leads to another, which then leads to another and another, and so on, therefore leading toward increasingly dark scenarios. Explain that when a person has such thoughts and is convinced of the power of positive thinking (after having read books on the subject, for example), they tend to conclude that they think too negatively and that they must therefore change all their negative thoughts into positive ones, such as: "This cancer will not get the best of me," "I will be cured," or "Cancer is a good thing, I will learn from it." Ask participants if they believe that positive thinking could help this person feel better. They will probably answer yes, so emphasize the fact that its effect is not long-lasting.

1.8.5   Slide #26: Effects of Positive Thinking

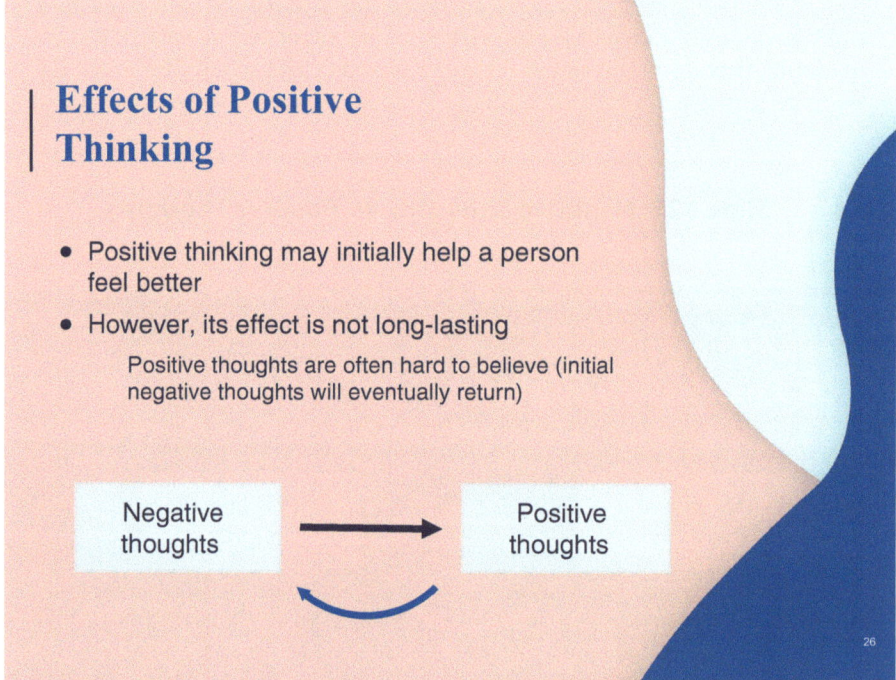

Though positive thoughts may initially block a negative reaction, they are often hard to believe. For example, a person finds out that a celebrity with a seemingly positive attitude died of cancer. The person might then tell themselves: "This could happen to me too." It is therefore quite likely that the initial negative thoughts will eventually return.

Continue the description of Melissa's case by mentioning the following to participants:

1.8 The Vicious Circle of the Tyranny of Positive Thinking: The Case of Melissa

Facilitator: In Melissa's mind, there is a perpetual battle going on between the negative thoughts that spontaneously emerge and the positive ones that she is trying very hard to maintain. In this mental battle, the negative thoughts often end up taking over because of their strong power. Saying to ourselves "I am going to die" is indeed a powerful thought. We can compare this battle to one between two boxers where one represents the negative thoughts with a strong and muscular body, and the other represents the positive thoughts with a smaller, much less strong body. At the start of the fight, the positive thoughts boxer will be able to withstand the blows that come from the negative thoughts boxer, but the former will eventually become exhausted because the latter is much more powerful. This mental battle ends up being very exhausting in the long run since it demands a lot of energy, which eventually causes the negative thoughts to take over.

Facilitator: In short, we have seen that positive thoughts can initially help reduce negative emotions. However, this effect does not tend to last because positive thoughts are often difficult to believe. As soon as a doubt emerges in our mind, the negative thoughts tend to return. Of course, our intention here is not at all to discourage you. We just want to point out that positive thinking may not be as magical as many people claim.

Possible question from participants

Participant: Can positive thinking be part of a person's nature?

Facilitator: Yes, absolutely!

Participant: I do not have to force myself to be positive. I was positive throughout my treatments, and I did not have to force it at all. It is just part of my personality.

Facilitator: There are indeed some people whose nature is more optimistic. No matter what the situation they encounter, they tend to see the positive side of things and expect that the future will hold more good than bad for them. For these people, no change is necessary. We do not need to change something that works well. Change is required when there is a perpetual mental battle where negative thoughts spontaneously take over due to their strength and power. We then try with all our might to be more positive even though this is not quite in our nature. As it happens, most people are not born optimists. As human beings, our ability to negatively anticipate the future and detect potential dangers in our environment has certainly helped our species survive. From the evolution of species perspective, this anticipation is considered adaptive, though it also has emotional consequences.

1.9 What Does Research Say About the Effects of Positive Thinking?

Section objectives:

- **Define dispositional optimism.**
- **Point out the connection between the different types of optimism (dispositional vs. unrealistic) and psychological distress in the context of cancer.**
- **Help participants understand that positive thinking does not seem to have the magical effect advocated by pop psychology books.**
- **Explain that the warrior metaphor often advocated by the positive thinking approach is appealing because of the false sense of control it provides, but can also cause feelings of guilt.**

Facilitator: So far, we have seen that studies do not show a link between mental attitude and cancer survival. But is it associated with a better adjustment to cancer? Many studies have focused on the effects of optimism.

1.9 What Does Research Say About the Effects of Positive Thinking?

1.9.1 Slide #27: Effects of Optimism

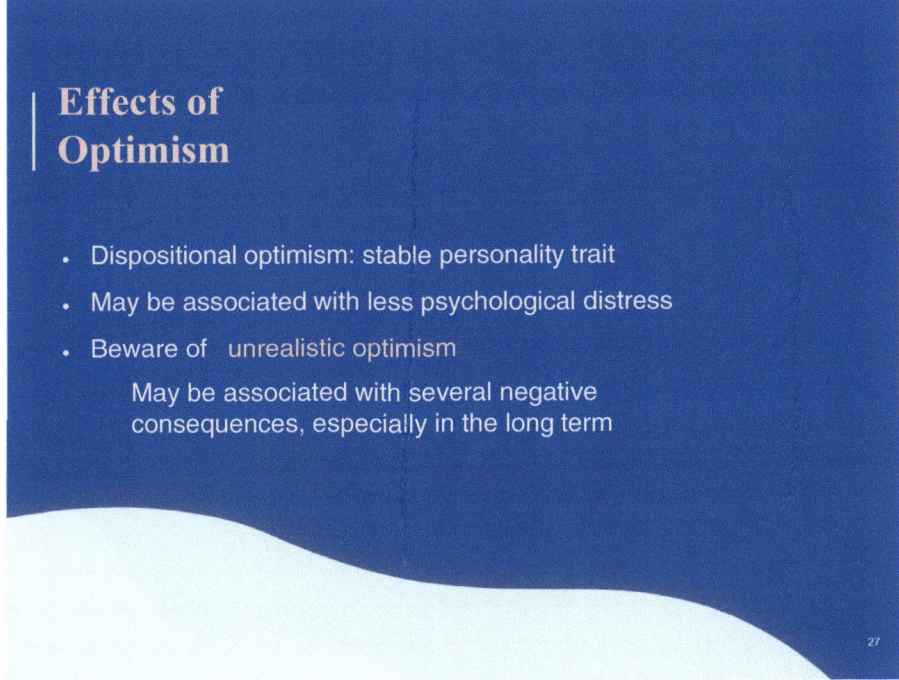

Explain that optimism is a personality trait that does not change much over a lifetime. Dispositional optimism is the tendency to expect that more positive than negative things will happen in our lives. Then, summarize the results of some studies that revealed that optimism is associated with experiencing less psychological distress in the context of cancer. However, point out that there are more and more indications in scientific literature that call for caution regarding unrealistic optimism.

> **Facilitator:** In a qualitative study carried out with patients with Parkinson's disease (Hurt et al., 2012), researchers found that optimistic patients experienced less depression right after receiving their diagnosis. However, once the disease had progressed, patients who were initially more optimistic had higher levels of depression compared to those whose initial reaction was more negative. In other words, having what could be described as unrealistic optimism at the time of diagnosis, and therefore thinking that everything will be fine, may protect a person psychologically in the short term. However, in the long run, this optimism is not helpful and can even hinder adjustment to the disease as it progresses. We must therefore keep this in mind and remain vigilant.

1.9.2 Slide #28: Fighting Cancer?

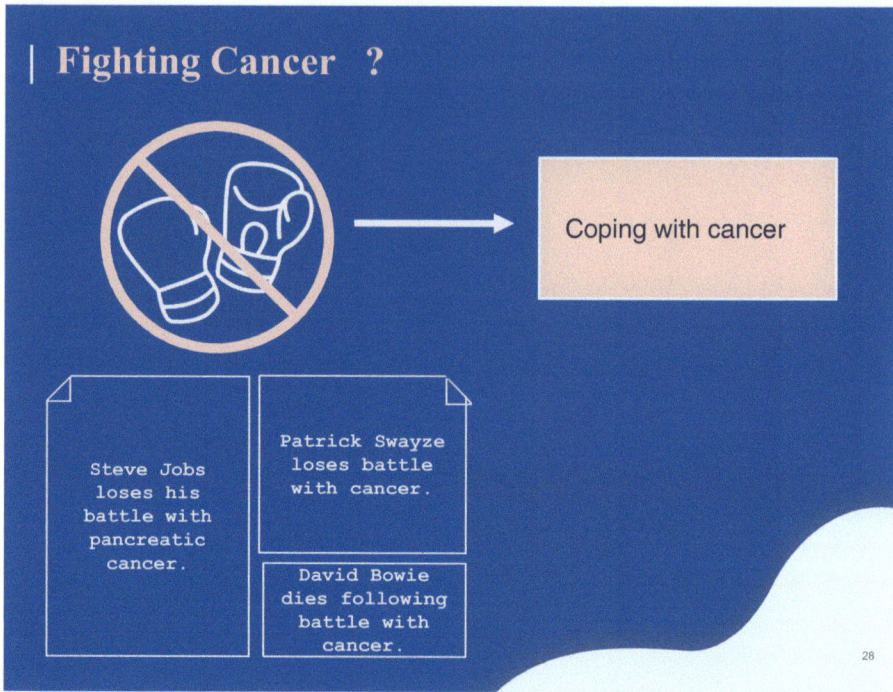

Facilitator: We will now talk about the warrior metaphor often advocated by the positive thinking approach, which can also be extremely guilt-inducing. We often hear that one must fight cancer: "Fight it, you will win the battle." We are very reluctant about this metaphor because, in a battle, there is always a winner and a loser. Newspapers regularly report news about celebrities who died from cancer: "Patrick Swayze loses battle with cancer," "David Bowie dies following battle with cancer," "Steve Jobs loses his battle with pancreatic cancer," etc. This type of news is very damaging because it puts a lot of responsibility on the ill person who is certainly not responsible for their disease's outcome. It also puts enormous pressure on people with cancer in general because they are not responsible for the way their cancer progresses. You may not experience this guilt personally, but it has been regularly observed in other people.

Facilitator: Cancer often generates a sense of loss of control over the disease, so the warrior metaphor may be used in an effort to regain a certain sense of control. But in reality, what does "Fighting cancer" really mean? What can we concretely do?

Participant: We can simply tell ourselves that we did our best by receiving the prescribed treatments. We can also consider what we can change in our life. For example, we can adopt healthier lifestyle habits. We can do our best, but this is not always enough.

Facilitator: Indeed, apart from receiving treatments and changing certain lifestyle habits to maximize our chances of being cured, we cannot do much else. Unless, of course, we claim we can fight cancer with positive thinking, but we have already seen how this can have negative consequences. All this stirs up a lot of guilt in people diagnosed with cancer, but also in those whose disease progresses. Instead, we suggest speaking in terms of "coping with cancer" rather than "fighting cancer."

Participant: People congratulate me. I tell them that I did not do anything. I got through it with a positive attitude, but my body did the actual work. I feel bad when people say such things to me. I feel bad for the others next to me for whom treatment did not work.

Facilitator: Exactly. However, I would not say that you did not do ANYTHING. For instance, you are responsible for the mental attitude you adopted toward the disease, the way you invested yourself in your treatments, and your lifestyle habits, which are all elements that may have helped your well-being and recovery. However, what you indeed had little power over was how the disease evolved in your body and responded to treatment. And if your body had not responded, you would have had nothing to do with it, and you would not have been a loser because of it.

1.10 The Benefits of Realistic Thinking

Section objectives:

- **Help participants see the difference between the different types of thoughts on the continuum.**
- **Illustrate the battle between negative and positive thoughts.**
- **Explain the concept of realistic thinking.**
- **Explain the main benefits of realistic thinking.**
- **Illustrate how realistic thinking can apply in the context of cancer.**

1.10.1 Slide #29: Dark Glasses vs. Rose-Coloured Glasses

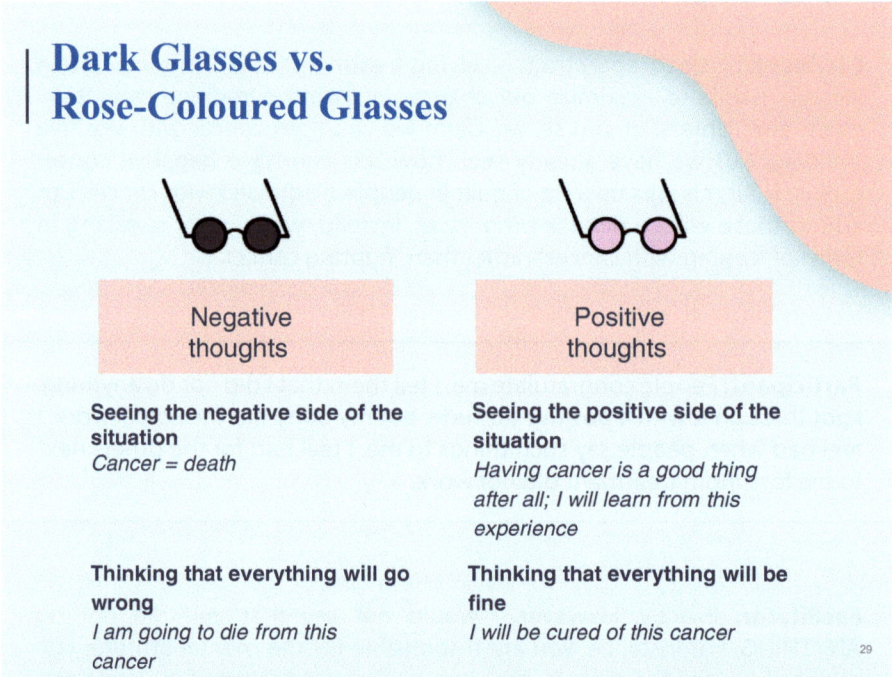

Show the participants the dark glasses image representing negative thoughts where situations that arise appear darker than they are. Then, show them the rose-coloured glasses image representing positive thoughts where the main focus is instead on the positive side of things and when we think that everything will be fine.

Next, explain the notion of the continuum of thoughts and introduce the concept of realistic thinking (Savard, 2010) as follows:

> **Facilitator:** When presented this way, it seems as though there are only two types of thoughts: positive and negative.

1.10 The Benefits of Realistic Thinking

1.10.2 Slide #30: Is There an Alternative?

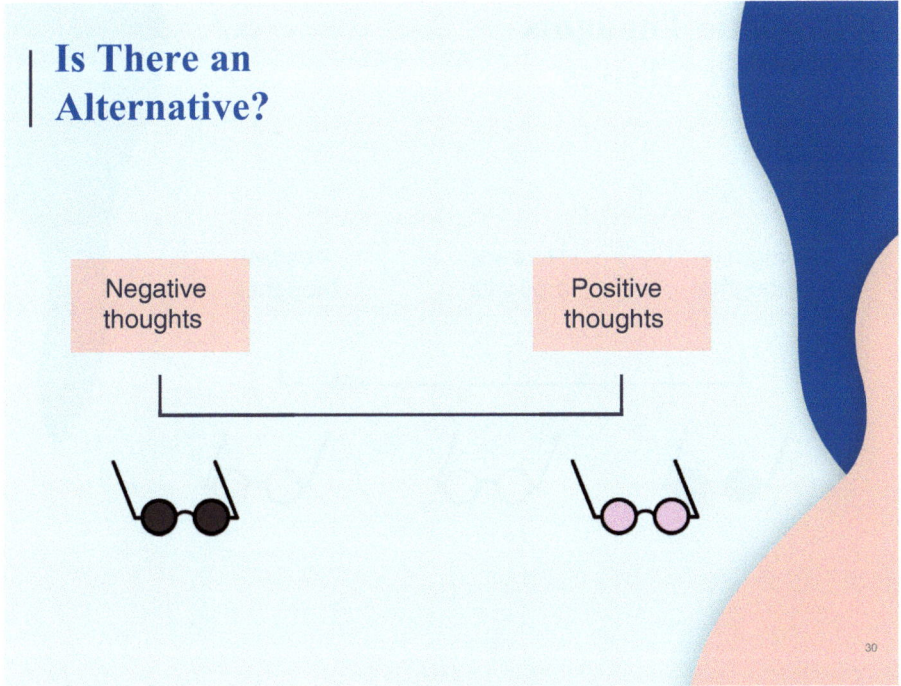

Facilitator: In reality, all the thoughts we have in a day, a week, or a year, are distributed along a continuum, ranging from very negative, which corresponds to the dark glasses, to very positive, as represented by the rose-coloured glasses.

1.10.3 Slide #31: Realistic Thoughts or Clear Glasses

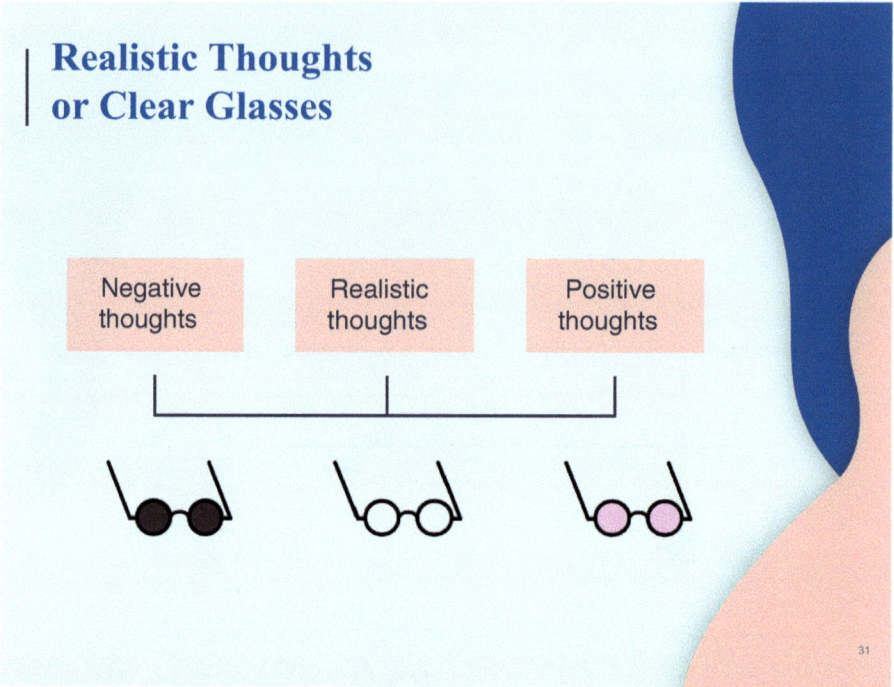

The continuum indicates that there is indeed an alternative in the middle: it is called realistic thinking and it is represented by clear glasses.

1.10.4 Slide #32: What Is Realistic Thinking?

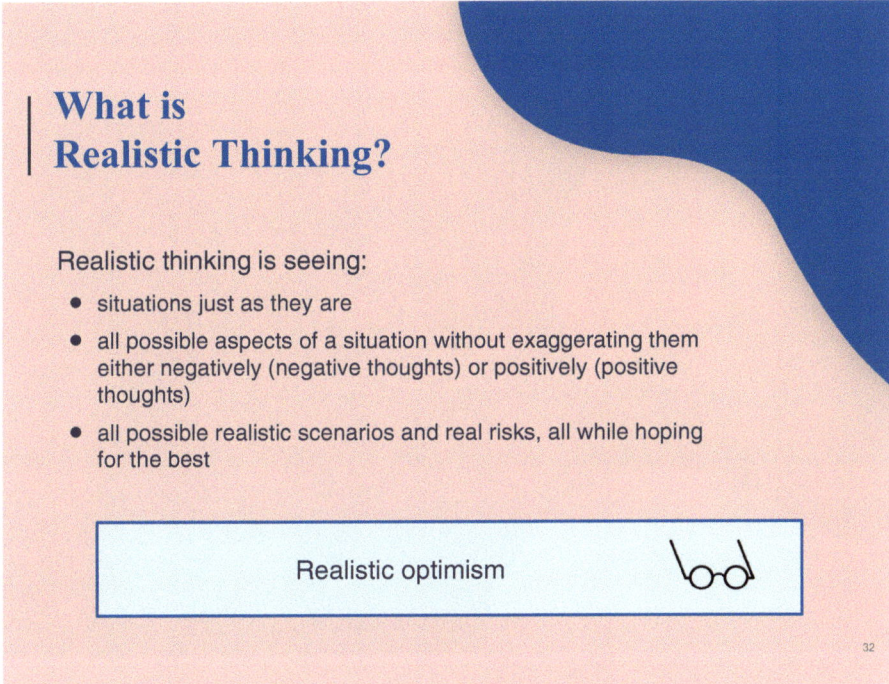

Facilitator: Realistic thinking is seeing situations that occur in our lives just as they are without exaggerating them positively, which would be like wearing rose-coloured glasses, or negatively, which would be like wearing dark glasses. With realistic thinking, all possible scenarios and real risks are considered, all while hoping for the best. This phrase ("all while hoping for the best") is crucial, and if you should have to remember only one thing from this session, it should be this one. What makes the positive thinking approach so appealing is its ability to give people hope. Having hope is extremely important in a situation like the one you have experienced. But there is no need to resort to extreme positive thinking. For this reason, this approach could also be called "realistic optimism." And it is this specific approach that we propose in this programme to help you cope better with fear of recurrence.

1.10.5 Slides #33–34: The Case of Mary

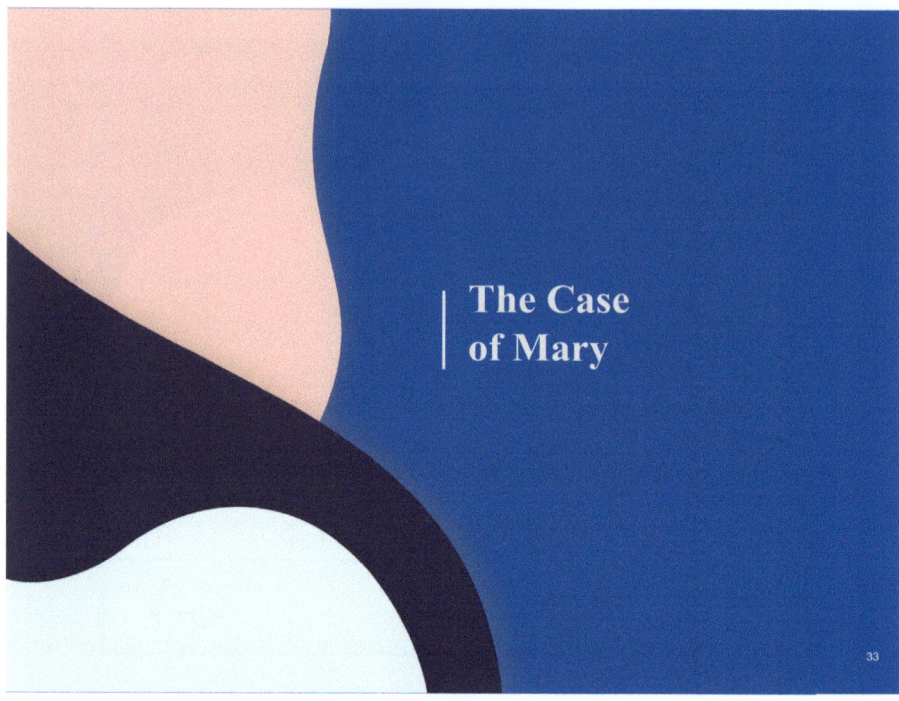

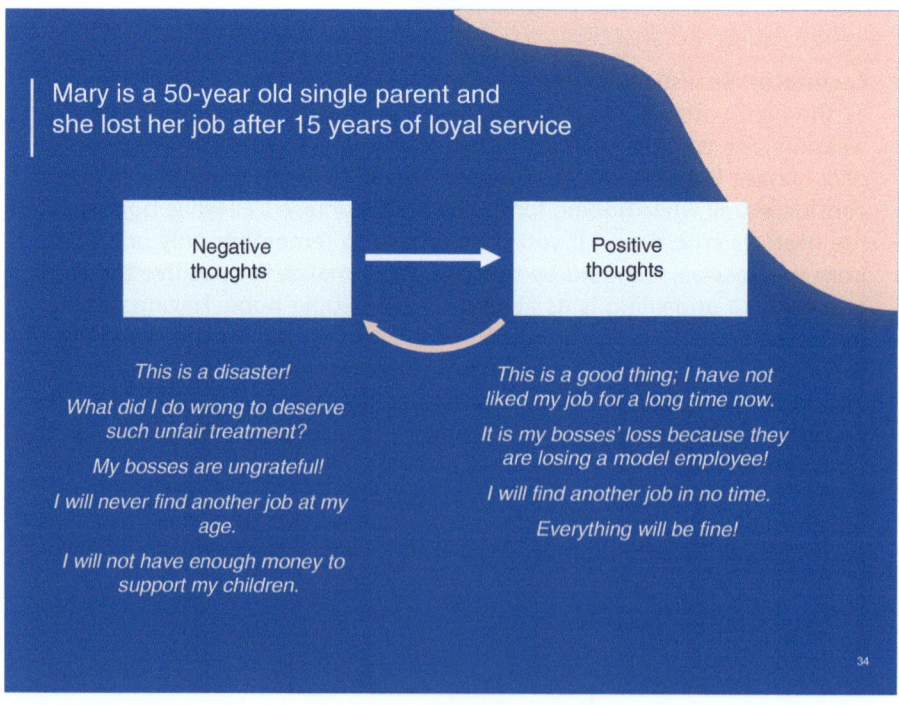

1.10 The Benefits of Realistic Thinking

Present the case of Mary to participants by mentioning the following:

> **Facilitator:** To practise realistic thinking, we will present the case of Mary, which is unrelated to cancer. Mary is 50 years old and a single parent. She lost her job after 15 years of loyal service and therefore finds herself in a very tough situation. At first, Mary had negative thoughts; she was wearing dark glasses, which is quite normal. What negative thoughts might Mary have in this scenario?

> **Participant:** I will not find another job.

> **Participant:** I am no good for anything anymore.

> **Participant:** It is my fault.

> **Participant:** I am going to have financial problems.

> **Facilitator:** Excellent! There are also other examples such as: "This is a disaster!" "What did I do wrong to deserve such unfair treatment?" "My bosses are ungrateful!" "I will never find another job at my age," or "I will not have enough money to support my children." We can see how her thoughts lead from one to another and ultimately become quite catastrophic. Therefore, Mary might consider thinking more positively as this could help her feel better. What positive thoughts (think in terms of rose-coloured glasses) could she try to have?

> **Participant:** There is something better out there waiting for me.

> **Facilitator:** Indeed, that is a good answer. She could also try telling herself: "This is a good thing because I have not liked my job for a long time now," "It is my bosses' loss because they are losing a model employee!" "I will find another job in no time," and "Everything will be fine!" As mentioned previously, "Everything will be fine" is often a positive thought we repeat to reassure ourselves. For a while, Mary may feel better, at least as long as she manages to maintain her positive thinking. But then, she could start to have doubts. For example, she could begin telling herself that it is not that easy to find a job at 50 and that she really needs another job quickly because her children depend on her. Then, what will happen? Probably what we described earlier: a mental battle will ensue, and the negative thoughts will end up taking over.

1.10.6 Slide #35: Mary and Realistic Thoughts

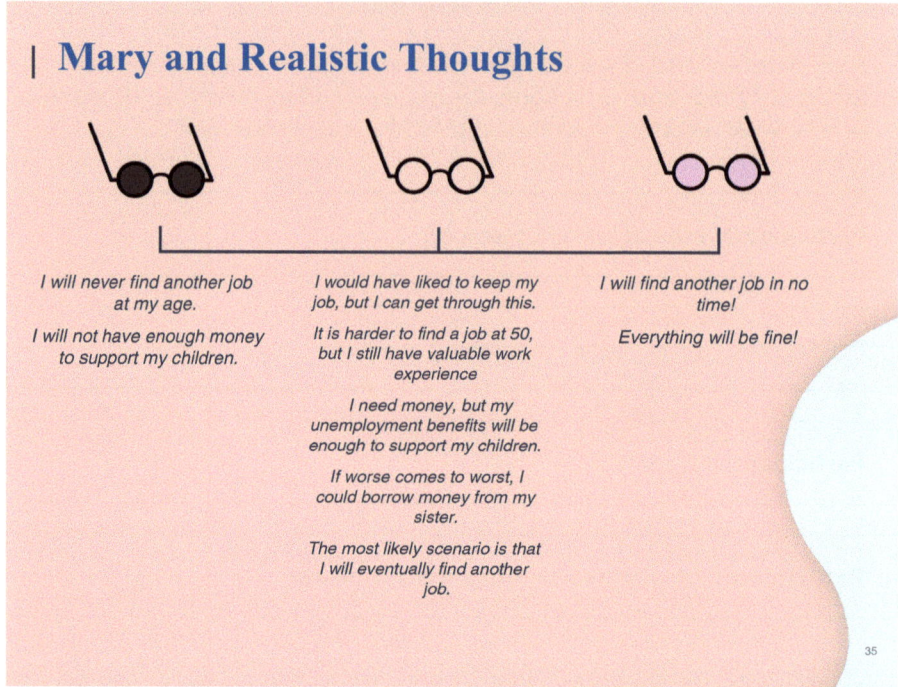

Facilitator: Now, let us see how we could help Mary better cope with her situation through realistic thinking. Initially, she had negative thoughts. She then tried to convince herself that everything would be fine. Now, remembering the definition of realistic optimism, which is imagining all the possible scenarios of a situation while hoping for the best, what realistic thoughts would be possible in Mary's situation?

Participant: I have 15 years of work experience, which may be appealing to a potential employer in the same field. I already have a certain degree of knowledge.

Facilitator: Excellent. With these thoughts, we are not at all in the positive thinking field and are not wearing rose-coloured glasses. She may indeed realize that she has valuable work experience and that a potential employer would probably consider this an asset.

1.10 The Benefits of Realistic Thinking

Participant: It is going to be tough, but I will manage to get through this.

Facilitator: Excellent!

Participant: This could be my chance to try something new, to make a career change.

Facilitator: Yes, that tends slightly toward positive thinking, but not too much. She could indeed turn her situation into an opportunity to make a career change. By the way, it is not necessary to be in the absolute middle of the continuum: thoughts can lean toward one side or the other (positive or negative thoughts) as long as they are not at the extremes.

Participant: If Mary gives her résumé to enough employers, she might be chosen by at least one of them.

Facilitator: Yes, that is a good observation, and it is also very realistic. We are not assuming that it will work every time, but out of all the résumés Mary gives to potential employers, she might get at least one job offer.

Participant: She could also establish a budget and find resources to help her with food and money.

Facilitator: Exactly! What you mentioned just now is vital. It is as if we asked ourselves: "What is the worst that could happen?" At this point, it is essential to consider all possible scenarios, even the worst ones. We can then ask ourselves if there are still solutions and if it would be possible to adjust to such a situation if it were to occur.

Facilitator: In short, Mary could recognize that she would have preferred to keep her job instead of trying to think positively by making herself believe that it is a good thing after all to have lost her job. In the end, she finally admits to herself that losing her job was bad news and that her situation is a challenging one, but she recognizes that she has the resources to make it through. Other possible realistic thoughts include: "I have faced other stressful events in my life and always managed to overcome them, so I should be able to overcome this one too," "It is indeed harder to find another job at 50, but I still have valuable work experience," "I do need money, but I get employment insurance benefits, and if worse comes to worst, I could always borrow money from my sister," or "I will most likely find another job sooner or later." Again, the idea is to consider all possible scenarios and hope for the best outcome.

1.10.7 Slide #36: Benefits of Realistic Thinking

Benefits of Realistic Thinking

- Reduces the strength and persistence of negative emotions
- Beneficial effect is longer lasting
- Helps find practical solutions and take action
- Helps to adjust to all possible consequences, even the worst ones

Summarize for participants the main benefits of realistic thinking compared to positive thinking. Tell them that it reduces the strength and persistence of negative emotions. Therefore, its beneficial effect is longer lasting compared to

1.10 The Benefits of Realistic Thinking   53

positive thinking that only works for a limited time. Moreover, explain that realistic thinking helps find practical solutions and take action, which is something that positive thinking does not allow for as much. Refer to Mary's case where she could, for example, update her résumé for a new job search, take training courses, apply for employment insurance benefits, ask her sister for help, and so on. Tell them that realistic thinking can also eventually help them adjust to all possible consequences by leading them to consider various scenarios, including even the worst ones, all while hoping for the best.

1.10.8   Slides #37–38: The Case of Louise

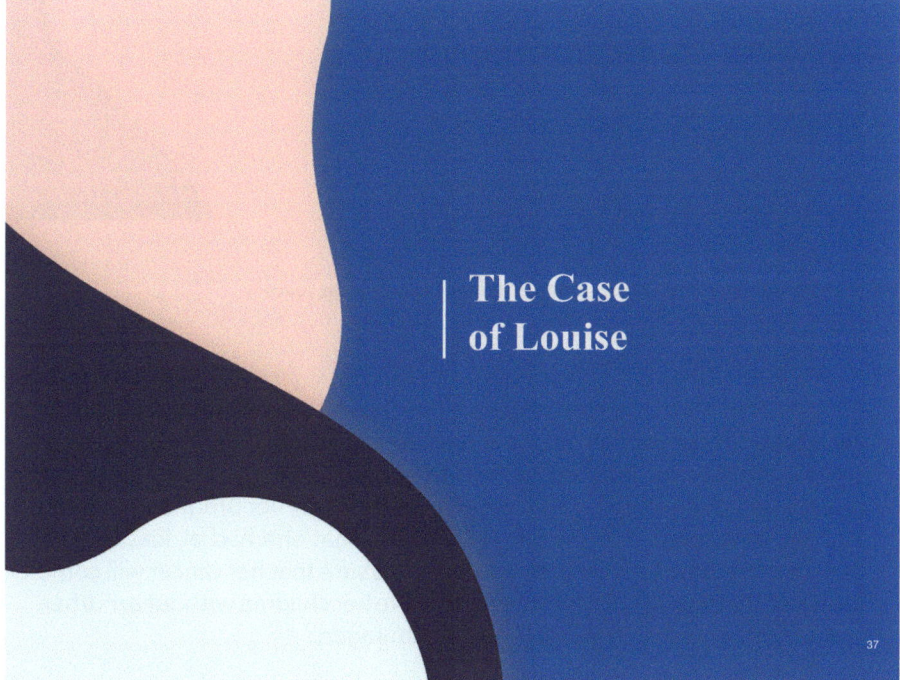

The Case of Louise

Louise just finished her treatments for ovarian cancer. Since her disease was discovered by chance, at an early stage, her prognosis is excellent. As it happens, her oncologist told her that she had at least a 95% chance of being cured. Despite this, Louise is sure that her cancer will come back and that she will die, which would leave her children without a mother.

Louise feels anxious, depressed, and discouraged.

Next, present the case of Louise, a cancer-related example, as follows:

Facilitator: Now, we will see how realistic thinking can apply in a cancer context. Louise just finished her treatments for ovarian cancer. Since her disease was discovered by chance, at an early stage, her prognosis is excellent. As it happens, her oncologist told her that she had at least a 95% chance of being cured. Despite this, Louise is sure that her cancer will come back and that she will die, which would leave her children without a mother. Louise feels anxious, depressed, and discouraged.

1.10.9 Slide #39: Cancer and Realistic Thoughts

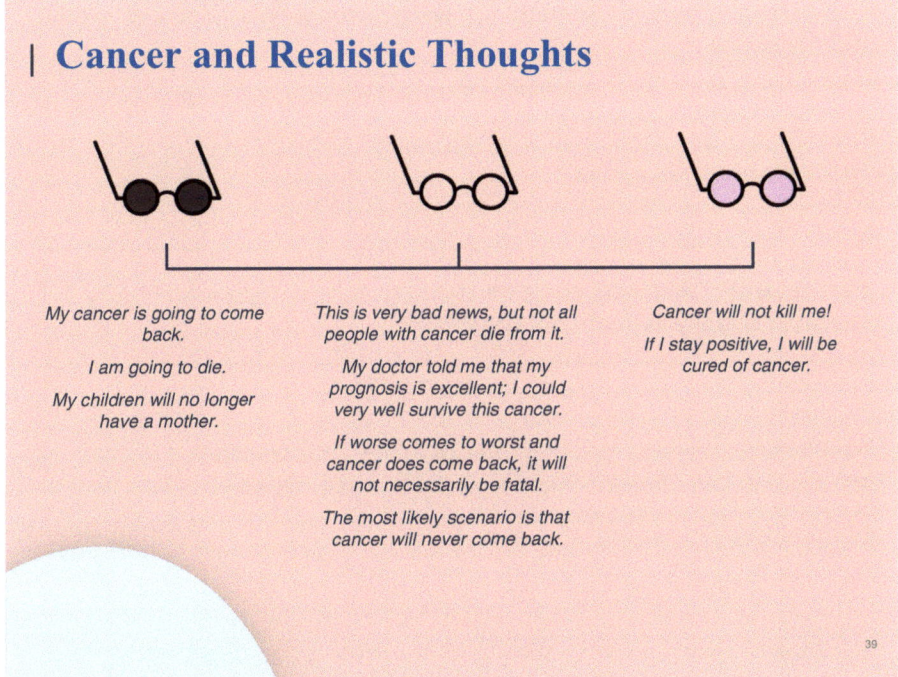

Facilitator: Earlier, we mentioned that the real risk of recurrence does not necessarily predict fear of recurrence intensity. Such is the case for Louise. She has much more chances of never having a cancer recurrence, but she is still quite worried about the other 5%. More specifically, her negative thoughts are: "My cancer is going to come back. I am going to die. My children are going to lose their mother." To lift her spirits, she could tell herself that she is too negative and try to be more positive. For example, she could try to convince herself that her cancer will not kill her and that she will be cured if she remains positive.

Facilitator: Now, what realistic thoughts would be suitable in this situation? Remember to consider all possible scenarios.

Participant: She could try telling herself that she is under the care of health professionals and if something were wrong, her doctors would quickly notice.

Facilitator: Yes, very good.

Participant: What most people tell themselves is: "It might come back," but we could also say "It might not come back."

Facilitator: Excellent! In that sentence alone, all scenarios are present. In the end, we can hope for the best possible outcome, which would be that cancer does not come back.

Facilitator: Here, Louise admits that her cancer is bad news, but she also recognizes that not all people with cancer die from it. Other realistic thoughts are: "My doctor told me that my prognosis is excellent," "If worse comes to worst and my cancer does come back, it does not necessarily mean that it will be fatal." This last statement is important because when we refer to cancer recurrence, we often instantly think of death as if it were automatically going to occur. As we will see in another session, cancer recurrence is not necessarily synonymous with death, much in the same way that cancer is not automatically synonymous with death. The most likely scenario is that Louise's cancer will never come back since she has a 95% chance of not having a recurrence.

At this point, ask participants whether they have comments, questions, or reactions to share.

1.11 Cognitive-Behavioural Therapy   57

1.10.10 Slide #40: Do You Need to Change Your Way of Seeing Things?

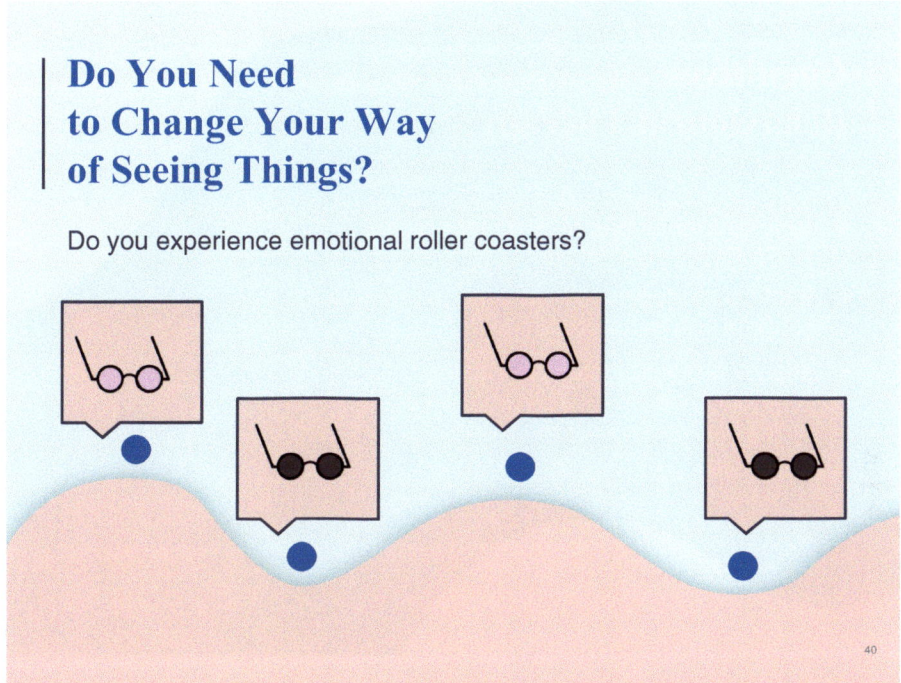

At this point, participants may be wondering whether it would be relevant for them to change their ways of coping with the disease. So, tell them that if they tend to experience emotional roller coasters, that is, if they tend to feel good as long as they manage to maintain positive thoughts, but their mood is affected when negative thoughts take over, and all this demands a lot of their energy, realistic thinking (i.e. moving closer to the middle of the continuum) would very likely be a good option for them.

1.11 Cognitive-Behavioural Therapy

Section objectives:

- **Explain what cognitive-behavioural therapy is along with its empirical support.**
- **Remind participants that it is impossible to guarantee that the proposed psychotherapy will be 100% effective for them and that the aim is to reduce their fear of recurrence in order to help them cope better with cancer.**

1.11.1 Slide #41: Cognitive-Behavioural Therapy

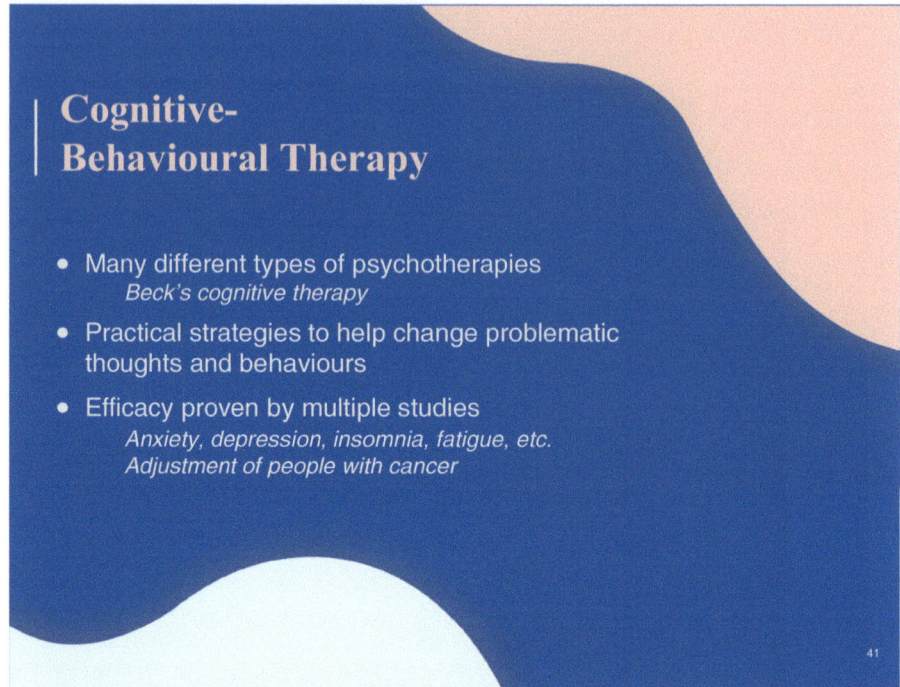

In this section, explain to participants the proposed therapy model. The approach recommended in this program is cognitive-behavioural therapy (CBT) and it includes many different types of psychotherapies. Tell them that it is primarily the cognitive therapy approach proposed by Dr Aaron T. Beck that we will be using in this group.

Next, explain to them in more detail what CBT is. Specify that the term "cognitive" in "cognitive-behavioural" refers to thoughts and interpretations and the "behavioural" part refers to the actions and behaviours that aim to help them adjust to events that occur. Then, explain that the basic principle of CBT is that thoughts play a primary role in the onset and persistence of emotions. Again, it is not the events in themselves that generate or maintain emotional reactions but rather their interpretation.

Also, mention to participants that CBT proposes practical strategies to help change thoughts and behaviours. Explain that they must first observe their thoughts and behaviours more closely, then they must identify those that seem problematic in order to try to change them. Mention that during the following sessions, different tools will be suggested to help them reach this goal.

Then, tell participants that CBT is a form of psychotherapy that has been proven effective in multiple studies and for various types of problems, such as anxiety, depression, and insomnia, both for the general population and people with cancer. However, it is essential to remind them that it is impossible to guarantee that this therapy will be 100% effective in their case. In short, the general goal of psychotherapy is to help people adjust better, and this is precisely the aim of this psychotherapy group.

1.12 Recognizing Negative Thoughts

Section objectives:

- **Help participants better recognize negative thoughts by describing their main characteristics.**
- **Point out that identifying negative thoughts and common cognitive distortions increases our awareness of them, which in turn makes them easier to change.**

1.12.1 Slide #42: Characteristics of Negative Thoughts

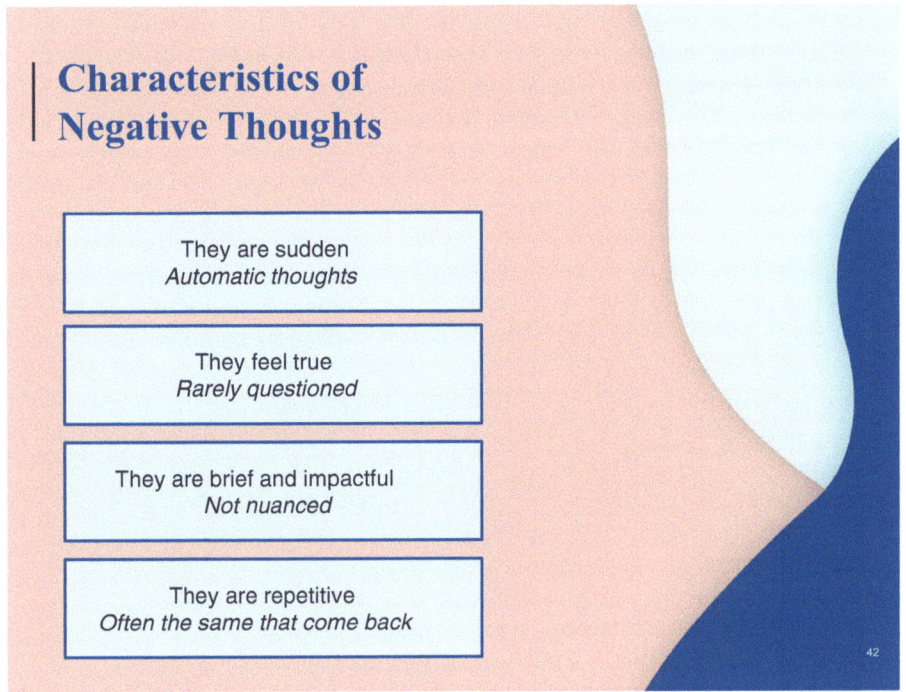

Tell participants about the different characteristics of negative thoughts in order to introduce the cognitive restructuring strategy, which will be presented in more detail in the next session.

> **Facilitator:** The first strategy that we are going to present is called "cognitive restructuring." It involves questioning the validity and usefulness of our thoughts and adopting more realistic ones. We will discuss this in more detail in the next session, but the first step toward changing our thoughts is learning to identify them. While this might seem simple, the process can actually be quite complicated. Why? Because our thoughts are automatic and sudden. They pop up in our minds without us noticing them. Our brains are thinking machines. In the last hour, you have had hundreds of thoughts. Some of them stick while others pass without us even realizing it. Therefore, it is essential to take the time to notice them so we can be aware of what we are thinking in various situations. For example, we can ask ourselves the following: "What was I saying to myself about that? What were my thoughts?" Negative thoughts are also brief and impactful. Generally, the first thoughts that come to mind in a stressful situation are not thoughtful and nuanced. They are much like the thoughts we discussed earlier: "I am going to die," "It is over for me," and "Life is not worth living anymore."

> **Facilitator:** Moreover, one of the most problematic characteristics of negative thoughts is that they can feel true to us. Therefore, one of our goals is to help you question your negative thoughts and not always take them for facts. Also, thoughts are generally repetitive, which means that we often tend to have the same types of thoughts in certain situations. Therefore, some people regularly find themselves having thoughts that lead them to feel guilt or anger, as if their glasses were gaining a particular tint. For some, this tint may be marine blue. For others, it may be purple or dark green. The point is that these different shades will make us see things from a different perspective. However, more often than not, a person will have the same types of cognitive distortions. Therefore, it is quite useful to learn to identify them because if, for example, we know that we always tend to think that things that happen are our fault, it will be easier to identify and modify this inner speech the next time it occurs.

1.13 Thought Identification Exercise

1.13.1 Slide #43: Identification of Negative Thoughts

Identification of Negative Thoughts

Situation	Automatic thoughts	Emotions
Report the facts without interpreting them	Note thoughts without censoring them (often a cascade of thoughts)	Note the intensity of the emotion felt (%)

Which thoughts or which images came to your mind in the

situation _____

when you felt _____

Beck (1995). Adapted and reproduced with the permission of the author and the publisher.

Explain the exercise for identifying negative thoughts that participants are encouraged to complete at home during the week. First, hand them out a sheet so they can follow the explanations for the exercise. The exercise aims to help them identify and recognize thoughts associated with unpleasant emotions and become more aware of situations where such thoughts and feelings tend to surface. Tell them that they do not have to write down the information by following the order in the grid because the negative emotion will often be the first noticeable sign that something is going on. Knowing this will make it easier for them to identify thoughts associated with their emotions along with the situation in which they occur. Tell them that the situation description refers only to the presentation of objective and uninterpreted facts.

When identifying their thoughts, they must also be able to do so without censoring them. Ideally, they should write them down immediately, as soon as they arise in their mind, while the situation is still ongoing. Next, give them an example with the grid to illustrate your explanations. It could be a person who is watching television and, by chance, comes across a report on cancer with testimonials from people who experienced a cancer recurrence (situation). Next, the person identifies the thoughts that come spontaneously to mind, for example: "It is going to happen to me too. My cancer is going to come back!" and notes the emotions associated with them, such as anxiety or sadness. It is also essential to record the intensity of the emotion by indicating a percentage, where 0 represents an absence of emotion and 100 represents the most intense emotion. This will be useful later on when cognitive restructuring is introduced.

Tell participants that the exercise should ideally focus on the thoughts they have about fear of cancer recurrence. However, if they do not experience a situation directly related to cancer over the next week, they can practice with other topics. Tell them that there will be a group discussion about the exercise at the start of the next meeting during which they may share what they learned if they wish to do so. In the end, the goal is to do the exercise for their own benefit.

1.13.2 Slide #44: Exercise to Do at Home

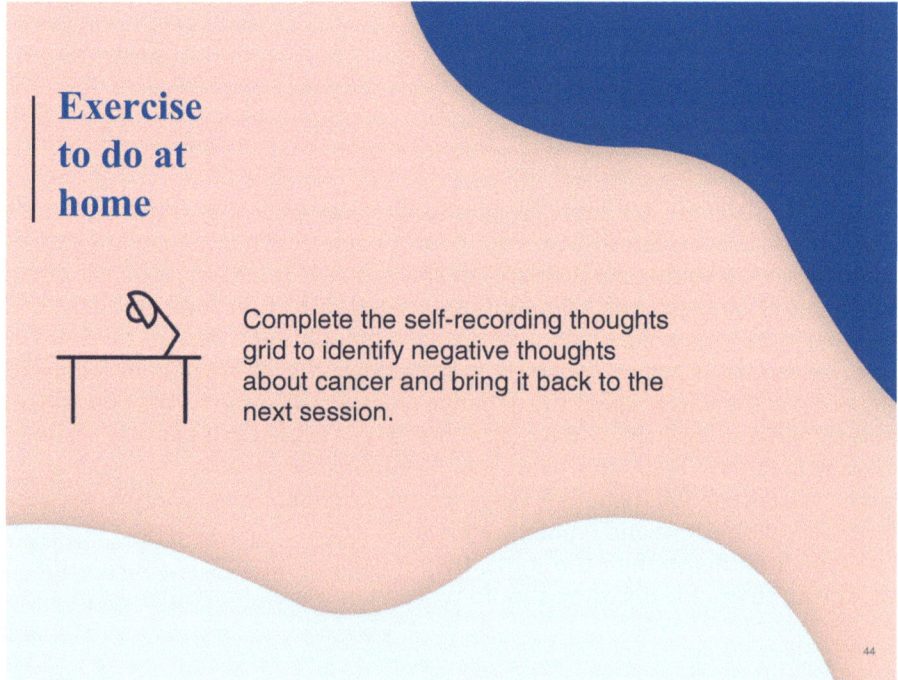

1.14 Slide #45: End of Session Discussion

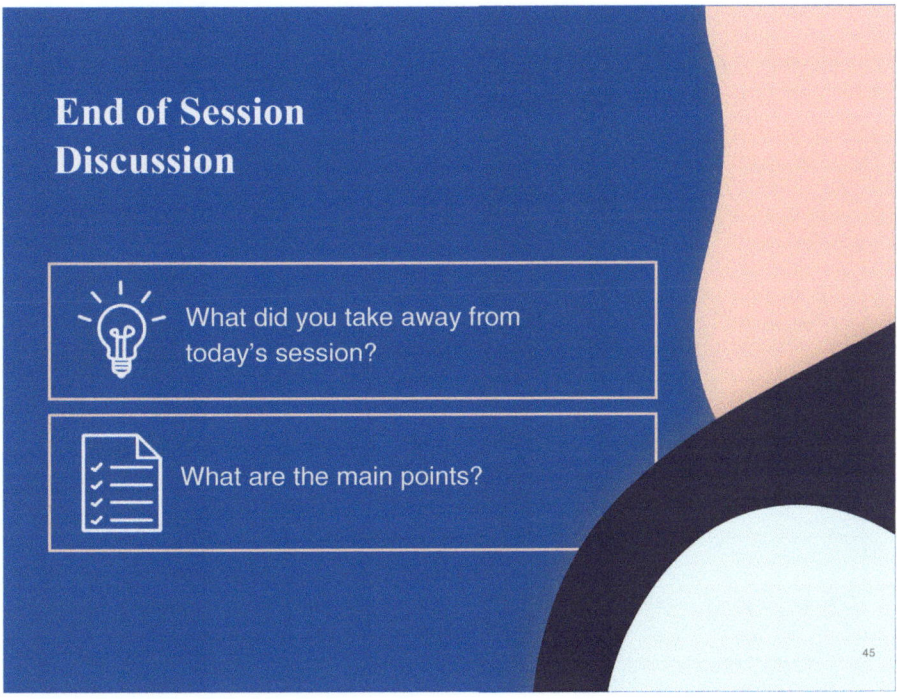

Ask participants what they took away from the session (2 to 4 main points). Survey their impressions, appreciation, and comments. Also, ask them if they have questions about the content of today's presentation.

1.15 Slide #46: Tools in Brief

Tools in Brief

Issues	Solutions
Endorsing beliefs that stress = cancer or positive thinking = cure	Discussion about the lack of scientific support for these ideas Multifactorial model of cancer Tyranny of positive thinking Understanding the effect of unrealistic optimism on adjustment to cancer
Tendency to alternate between positive thoughts (hard to believe) and negative thoughts (associated with distress)	Analogy of dark glasses and rose-coloured glasses Understanding that thoughts are on a continuum Alternative of clear glasses that represent realistic thinking
Difficulty recognizing one's thoughts	Understanding that negative thoughts are sudden, brief and powerful, that they seem true and are repetitive Identification of negative thoughts exercise

Summarize the main strategies discussed during the session for dealing effectively with certain issues related to fear of recurrence.

References

Coyne, J. C., Ranchor, A. V., & Palmer, S. C. (2010). Meta-analysis of stress-related factors in cancer. *Nature Reviews, 7*, 1–2.

Dumalaon-Canaria, J. A., Prichard, I., Hutchinson, A. D., & Wilson, C. (2018). Fear of cancer recurrence and psychological well-being in women with breast cancer: The role of causal cancer attributions and optimism. *European Journal of Cancer Care, 27*(1).

Goodwin, P. J., et al. (2001). The effect of group psychosocial support on survival in metastatic breast cancer. *The New England Journal of Medicine, 345*, 1719–1726.

Hurt, C. S., Weinman, J., Lee, R., & Brown, R. G. (2012). The relationship of depression and disease stage to patient perceptions of Parkinson's disease. *Journal of Health Psychology, 17*, 1076–1088.

Lebel, S., Ozakinci, G., Humphris, G., et al. (2016). From normal response to clinical problem: Definition and clinical features of fear of cancer recurrence. *Support Care Cancer, 24*, 3265–3268.

References

Olsen, M. H., Nielsen, H., Dalton, S. O., & Johansen, C. (2015). Cancer incidence and mortality among members of the Danish resistance movement deported to German concentration camps: 65-Year follow-up. *International Journal of Cancer, 136*, 2476–2480.

Pedersen, A. F., Rossen, P., Olesen, F., von der Maase, H., & Vedsted, P. (2012). Fear of recurrence and causal attributions in long-term survivors of testicular cancer. *Psycho-Oncology, 21*, 1222–1228.

Savard, J. (2010). *Faire face au cancer avec la pensée réaliste*. Montréal: Flammarion Québec.

Savard, J., Savard, M.-H., Caplette-Gingras, A., Casault, L., & Camateros, C. (2018). Development and feasibility of a group cognitive-behavioral therapy for fear of cancer recurrence. *Cognitive and Behavioral Practice, 25*, 275–285.

Spiegel, D., Bloom, J. R., Kraemer, H. C., & Gottheil, E. (1989). Effect of psychosocial treatment on survival of patients with metastatic breast cancer. *Lancet, 2*, 888–891.

Session No. 2

Structure of Session No. 2

Section title	Learning objectives	Page
Session agenda	• Present the topics that will be discussed during the session.	68
Review of the previous session	• Review the highlights of the previous session (negative thoughts are associated with higher distress, positive thoughts can be comforting, but only in the short term and cause feelings of anxiety and guilt, alternative option = realistic optimism).	69
Review of last week's exercise	• Invite participants to share their experience. • If needed, present the bike or hockey coach analogy to remind participants of the importance of doing the proposed exercises.	70
Cognitive restructuring	• Define and explain cognitive restructuring. • Present the Socratic questioning process as a way to question the validity of their thoughts. • Demonstrate the technique with an exercise (the case of Elise). • Emphasize the importance of considering the worst-case scenario.	72
Interpreting physical symptoms	• Present the two most extreme types of attitudes regarding physical symptoms and their interpretation (negligence and hypervigilance). • Present the four objective criteria for evaluating physical symptoms and give examples for each of them.	81
Information-seeking profiles	• Present the two most common information-seeking profiles along with their impacts on anxiety. • Highlight the importance of seeking the amount of information with which they feel comfortable.	86

Supplementary Information: The online version contains supplementary material available at [https://doi.org/10.1007/978-3-031-07187-4_2].

Section title	Learning objectives	Page
Being well informed	• Identify reliable sources of information. • Suggest strategies for preparing for medical appointments.	89
Interpreting probabilities and statistics	• Explain what a statistic is and what some types of probabilities mean (risk of recurrence, five-year net survival rate, reduced risk of recurrence). • Emphasize that the actual risk of recurrence is not proportional to the level of anxiety felt and that statistics are constantly changing.	91
Cognitive restructuring exercise	• Propose and explain a cognitive restructuring exercise to do at home.	98
End of session discussion	• Ask participants what they took away from the session. • Answer questions and summarize key concepts as needed.	101

2.1 Session Agenda

2.1.1 Slide #3: Session No. 2

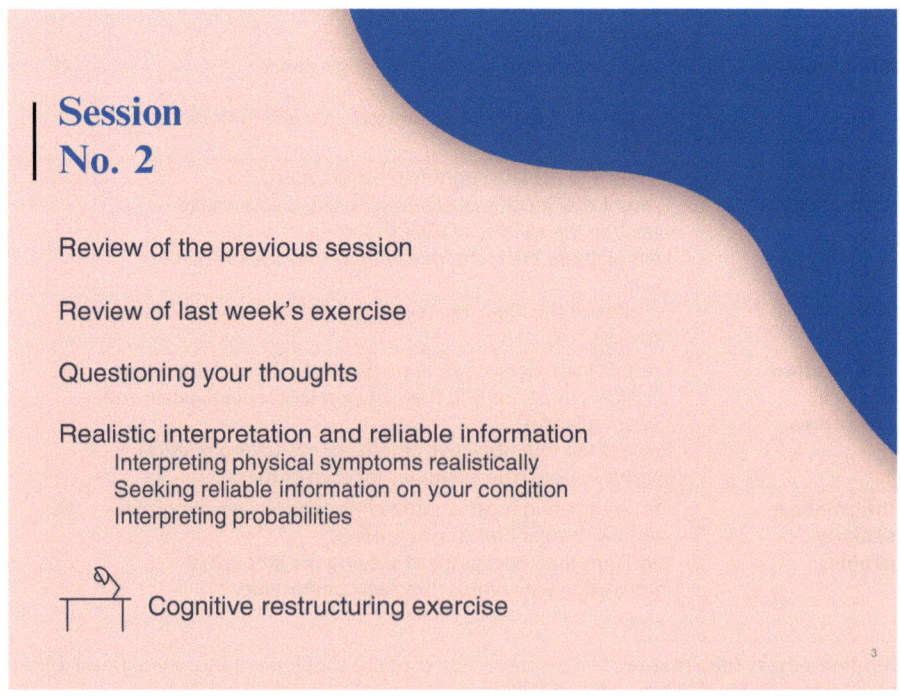

First, present the agenda for the session to participants:

- **Review of the previous session**
- **Review of last week's exercise**
- **Questioning your thoughts**
- **Realistic interpretation and reliable information**
  - Interpreting physical symptoms realistically
  - Seeking reliable information on your condition
  - Interpreting probabilities
- **Cognitive restructuring exercise**

2.2 Review of the Previous Session

Before delving into the content of this session, ask participants if they have any comments, questions, or thoughts they would like to share about the previous session. Ask them what the highlights of the last session were. Remind them that negative thoughts are generally associated with more psychological distress, and while positive thoughts may be comforting in the short term, they often have the adverse effect of stirring up feelings of guilt and anxiety because it is impossible to remain positive all the time. Realistic thinking (or realistic optimism) is a good alternative that is generally more effective in the long term. Tell them that the purpose of this session is to show them how to apply realistic optimism by changing their negative thoughts into more realistic ones.

2.3 Review of Last Week's Exercise

2.3.1 Slide #4: Review of the Thought Identification Exercise

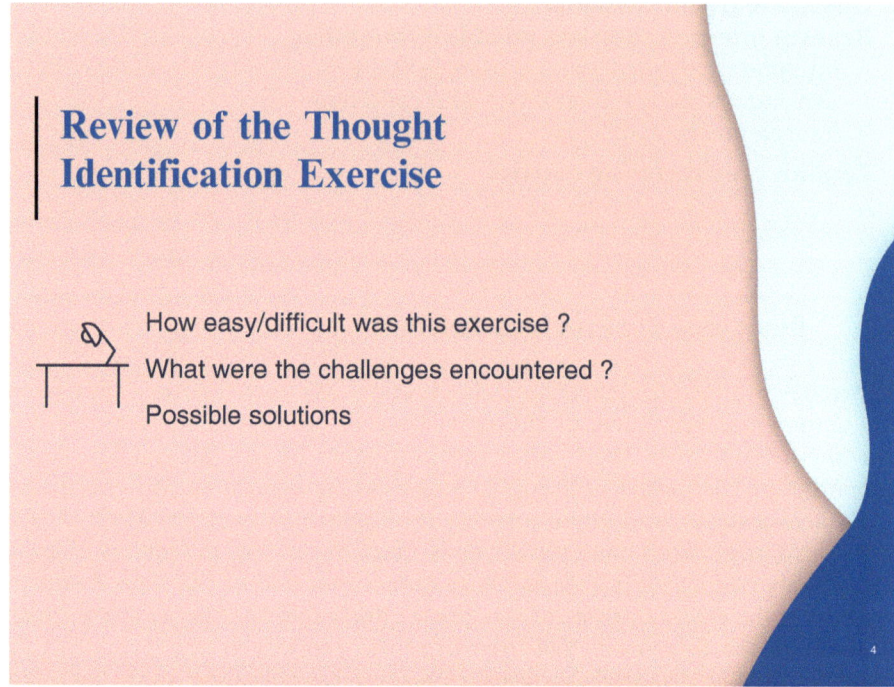

Discuss the exercise that was proposed at the end of last week's session. Ask if anyone would like to share their experience with the group. Next, ask them if doing the exercise (i.e. sorting into columns the situations, thoughts, and emotions related to a situation) was a challenge for them. You can also tell them that they may see you during the break if they have any questions about the exercise and do not feel comfortable asking them in front of the other participants or if they would like to receive more personal feedback regarding their situation. If necessary, reiterate the importance of doing the suggested exercises by using the bike analogy (i.e. the more we practice, the more skilful we become). To stress even further the importance of investing themselves in psychotherapy, you can also use the hockey coach analogy. Psychotherapy involves teamwork where the therapist can be seen as the coach and patients as the players. Despite all the encouragement and strategies that coaches can offer to help the players improve their game, they cannot score goals or block opponents' shots for them. Therefore, it is up to the players/patients, to use the suggested strategies to improve their game/way of dealing with their fear of cancer recurrence.

2.4 Fear of Cancer Recurrence Model

2.4.1 Slide #5: The Vicious Circle of Fear of Recurrence

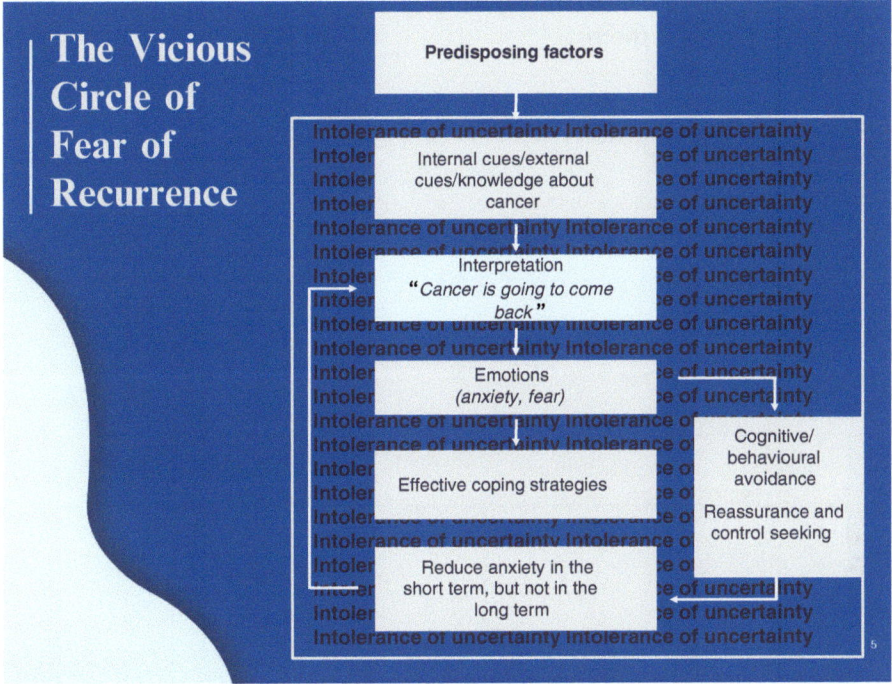

Present the fear of cancer recurrence model and specify that this session will again focus on the "Interpretation" box.

2.5 Cognitive Restructuring

Section objectives:

- Allow participants to practise identifying their negative thoughts and associated emotions as seen in the first session.
- Show them how to change their negative thoughts into realistic ones using the Socratic questioning method and cognitive restructuring technique, as illustrated in a clinical example (the case of Elise).
- Stress the importance of considering all possible scenarios (including the worst one).
- Reiterate the importance of doing exercises in writing and present the goal of cognitive restructuring (to help make emotions less overwhelming, not eliminate them).

2.5.1 Slide #6: Cognitive Restructuring Grid

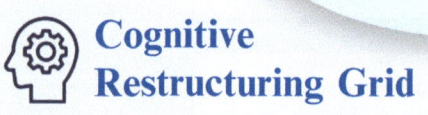

Situation	Negative thoughts	Emotions (%)	Realistic thoughts	Emotions (%)

Beck (1995). Adapted and reproduced with the permission of the author and the publisher.

Present the cognitive restructuring technique to participants. Explain that in the previous session and in the exercise they did at home, they learned to identify their negative thoughts, the situations in which they occur, and the emotions associated with them. In this session, they will learn how to change their negative thoughts into more realistic ones by applying the cognitive restructuring technique, that is, by questioning the validity of their thoughts. By changing their thoughts, the associated negative emotions will decrease.

2.5.2   Slide #7: The Case of Elise

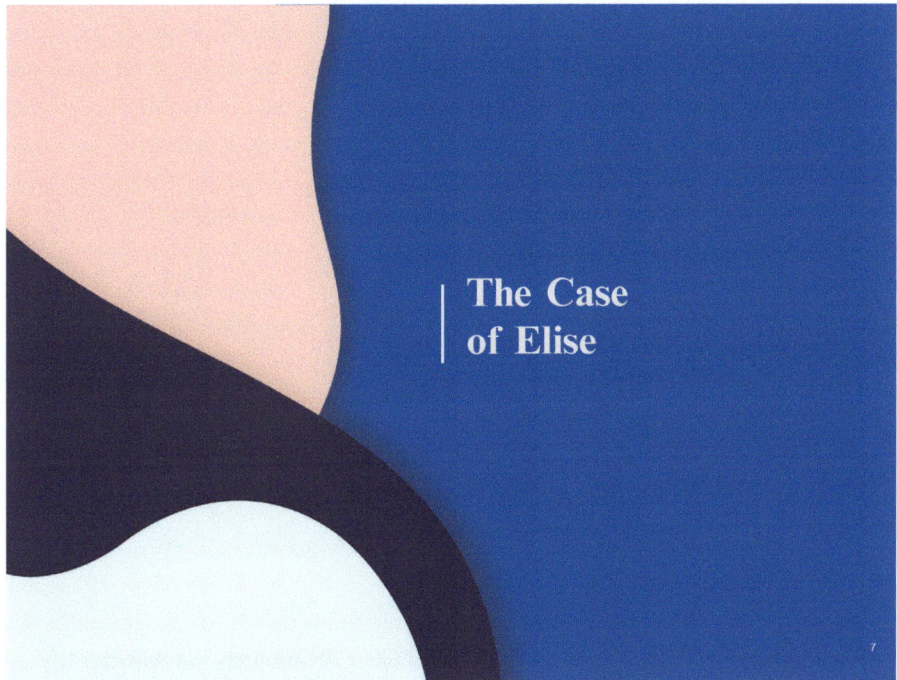

Next, do a cognitive restructuring exercise with the participants by presenting the case of Elise.

2.5.3 Slide #8: Fear of Recurrence

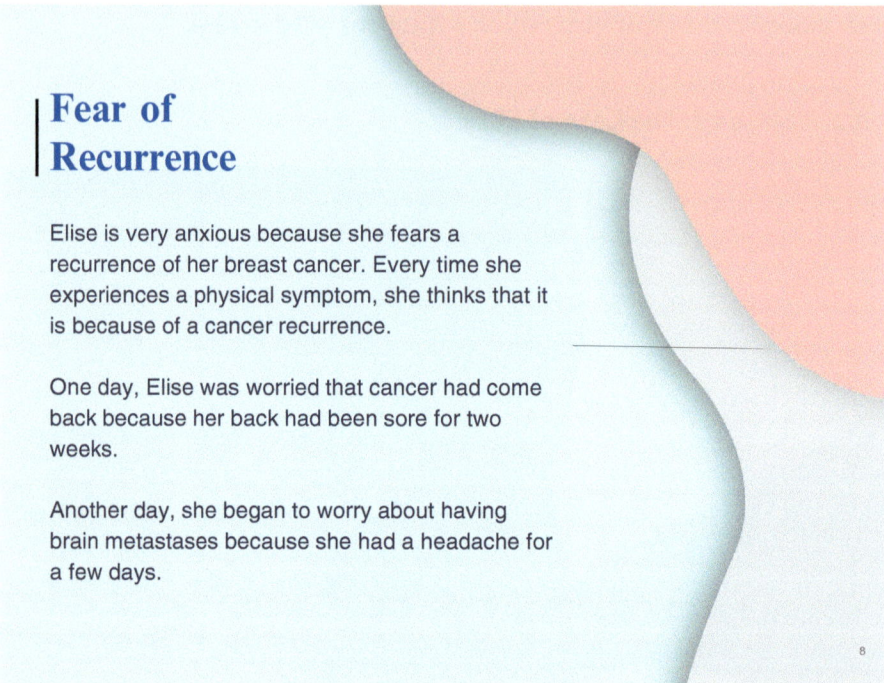

Facilitator: First, let's examine the case of Elise. Afterwards, we will identify thoughts and emotions that could be associated with her situation. We often present breast cancer examples because it is the most common form of cancer in women, but what we explain here applies to all types of cancer. So, here it is: Elise is very anxious because she fears a recurrence of her breast cancer. Every time she experiences a physical symptom, she thinks that it is because of a cancer recurrence. One day, Elise was worried that cancer had come back because her back had been sore for two weeks. Another day, she began to worry about having brain metastases because she had a headache for a few days. Based on what we have seen so far, what do you think Elise's negative thoughts and emotions would be?

Participant: "Has cancer come back?"

2.5 Cognitive Restructuring

Facilitator: Or: "This is it, it's back." Something like that.

Participant: "If cancer has come back, am I going to make it through again? Is this the end for me? Brain metastases are not operable. I'm going to die."

Facilitator: Yes, all those thoughts are very likely. And how is Elise likely to feel in response to these thoughts?

Participant: Anxious, depressed.

Facilitator: Yes, indeed.

2.5.4 Slide #9: The Case of Elise

Cognitive restructuring grid: The case of Elise

The Case of Elise

Situation	Negative thoughts	Emotions	Realistic thoughts	Emotions
I've had a headache for the past few days.	"I must have brain metastases." "I won't make it through the winter."	Anxious (100%) Depressed (80%)		

2.5.5 Slide #10: Questioning Your Thoughts

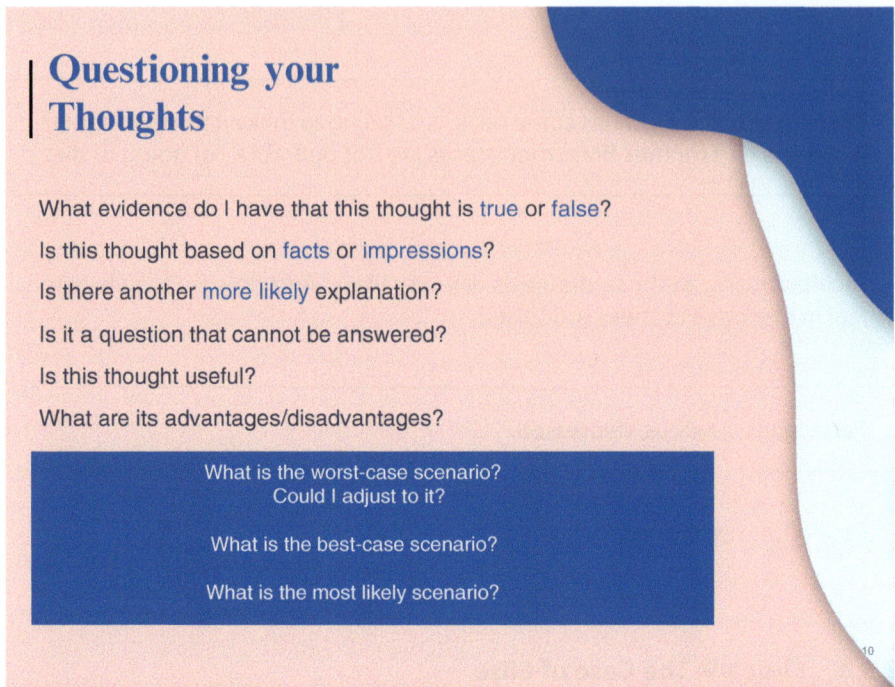

Next, present the Socratic questioning process. It involves questioning the validity of negative thoughts by asking yourselves various questions about them and exploring other possible interpretations to gain a more realistic view of the situation. Here are some examples of questions:

What evidence do I have that this thought is true? Or that it is false?
- **Is this thought based on facts or impressions?**
- **Is there another more likely explanation?**
- **What is the worst-case scenario, and could I adjust to it? What is the best-case scenario? What is the most likely scenario?**

- **Is it a question that cannot be answered?**
- **Is this thought useful? What are its advantages/disadvantages?**

> **Facilitator:** Because realistic optimism involves considering all possible scenarios, it is essential to ask yourselves what is the worst that could happen even if you find this difficult and unpleasant. "If the worst-case scenario were to occur, how could I adjust to it?" Conversely, what would be the best-case scenario? And among all these possible outcomes, which one would be the most likely and realistic? Of course, it is not always easy or pleasant to imagine the worst-case scenario, and we will come back to this later, but it is important to do so.

Go back to Elise's case and ask participants which questions she could ask herself to challenge the validity of her negative thoughts. Help them in this task by asking them if they have any other ideas or thoughts. Remind them of the definition of realistic optimism, which is to consider all possible scenarios, including the worst one, while still hoping for the best. Here are several examples of answers they may offer, along with potential feedback you could give them for each:

- Do headaches only occur when we have cancer, or can they also occur in other contexts? Tell participants that it is indeed relevant to consider alternative explanations and ask them what these explanations could be (e.g. stress, injury, etc.).
- If she made it through once, could she make it through again? Tell them that this is indeed a possible scenario and a very realistic one, too.
- What is the worst that could happen? Stimulate their thoughts on this particular question by asking them what it would mean if it were indeed a metastatic recurrence? Would this mean that she would die in the near future? The presence of metastases is not necessarily fatal: they can be treated, and many patients survive for years after being diagnosed with metastatic cancer. Remind them that other possible scenarios exist and that it is essential to ask themselves which one is the most likely.

2.5.6 Slide #11: The Case of Elise

The Case of Elise

Situation	Negative thoughts	Emotions	Realistic thoughts	Emotions
I've had a headache for the past few days.	"I must have brain metastases." "I won't make it through the winter."	Anxious (100%) Depressed (80%)	"I usually have this kind of pain a few days a month. It's probably just a normal headache." "My latest test results didn't reveal any signs of cancer." "The more I worry about my headache, the more likely it is to get worse." "If my headache persists or worsens, I will see my doctor to make sure that everything is fine." "The worst that could happen is finding out that I have metastatic cancer. It would be tough news to take; I would be devastated. However, there are treatments for metastases, and I would not necessarily die within the year." "The most likely scenario is that my headaches have nothing to do with cancer."	Anxious (30%) Depressed (20%)

Next, say the following to participants about realistic thoughts in Elise's case:

> **Facilitator:** After using the Socratic questioning technique, Elise came up with the following realistic thoughts: "I usually have this kind of pain a few days a month. It might just be a normal headache." "My latest results did not reveal any signs of cancer." Based on this factual information, her headache is unlikely to be due to cancer. Also, the more Elise worries about her headache, the more likely it is to get worse. Indeed, when we focus on a physical symptom, it tends to become worse. Of course, if her headache persists or worsens, she should see a doctor to make sure that everything is fine. "The worst that could happen is finding out that I have metastatic cancer. It would be tough news to take; I would be devastated. However, there are treatments for metastases and I would not necessarily die within the year." "The most likely scenario is that my headaches have nothing to do with cancer." "There are other possible scenarios, but the latter is the most likely."

2.5 Cognitive Restructuring

At this point, ask participants why they think Elise's anxiety and depression are not at 0% after she came up with more realistic thoughts. One correct answer is that anxiety and depression are not at 0% because there is always a level of uncertainty that remains when cancer is involved.

> **Facilitator:** The goal of cognitive restructuring is not to eliminate negative emotions or uncertainty. The fact is that we are discussing a sensitive issue, so it is normal to feel some degree of emotion. Instead, the goal is to make your emotions less overwhelming and thoughts less uncontrollable, and help you feel a greater sense of control over them. In Elise's example, we saw that her emotions significantly decreased, which means that the cognitive restructuring technique worked well.

Possible question from participants:

> **Participant:** Is it normal that I manage to reassure myself for a while, but that the emotion ends up coming back just as strong as before?

> **Facilitator:** As we saw last week, it may be because you practice positive thinking (e.g. telling yourselves that everything will be fine) to reassure yourself, but this strategy is only effective in the short term. Certainty that cancer will never come back is the only thing that would completely reassure you, but nobody can guarantee that. Cognitive restructuring, through which we identify all possible scenarios, while hoping for the best, has a more lasting effect but its goal is not necessarily to reassure you as such.

Next, remind participants that it is important to do the cognitive restructuring exercises in writing, especially when beginning to use this strategy. Explain that doing so will allow them to take a step back and put thoughts that are sometimes unclear into words, especially those that they tend to escape or avoid. Tell them that worries are often vague thoughts and will remain so unless they examine them more closely. Also, writing down realistic thoughts gives them more weight and effect than when they only try to identify them mentally. When the same negative thoughts arise again, they could read what they previously wrote down and avoid doing the exercise again from the start, hence allowing them to achieve a positive effect more quickly. Finally, tell them that they will have to do this type of exercise during the next week.

2.5.7 Slide #12: Recurrence ≠ Death

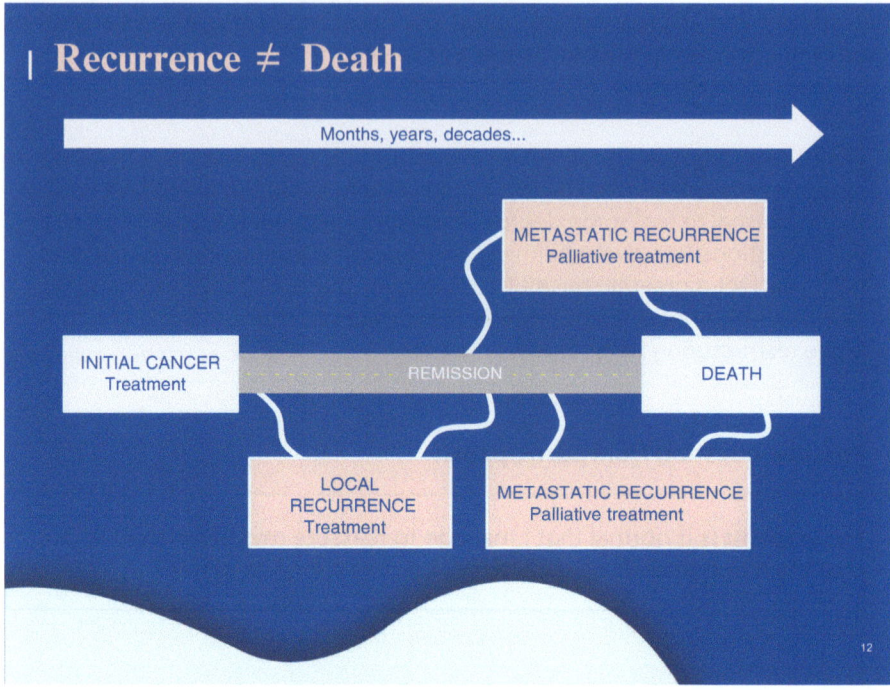

Facilitator: As we have just seen, when you are worried about cancer recurrence, it is crucial to remember that recurrence does not necessarily mean death. The only thing we know for sure is that we are all on a one-way road to death. Indeed, we are all going to die someday. However, we must not forget that many different paths can lead us to this outcome. Of course, if you had cancer before, the worst scenario and the most feared path is a metastatic recurrence that will rapidly lead to death. Emotionally, this is the most difficult scenario to think about. However, without denying it as a possibility, you must remember that there are still plenty of other possible paths. First, cancer might not come back, and you could die from some other cause. You could also develop, in a more or less near future, a local recurrence that can be treated effectively, and cancer might never come back again. Some people may develop several local recurrences and end up dying of other causes than cancer. Some patients could develop a metastatic recurrence in the near future or after several years, receive palliative treatment and have a good quality of life for many years before dying of cancer. Finally, a very catastrophic and possible scenario is a metastatic recurrence for which palliative treatment is ineffective and which would rapidly lead to death. However, remember that it would be a shame to consider only one scenario, especially the worst one, and worry about it excessively when there are many other possible scenarios that leave room to hope for the best possible outcome.

At this point, ask participants if they have any questions or comments about what has been discussed so far.

2.6 Interpreting Physical Symptoms

Section objectives:

- **Show participants how to interpret their physical symptoms more realistically.**
- **Present the two most extreme attitudes towards physical symptoms (negligence and hypervigilance) and their respective consequences.**
  - Explain the link between hypervigilance and fear of cancer recurrence.
- **Present the four objective criteria (NILP) to assess physical symptoms and give examples for each one:**
  - Novelty
  - Intensity
  - Likelihood
  - Persistence

2.6.1 Slide #13: Interpreting Physical Symptoms Realistically

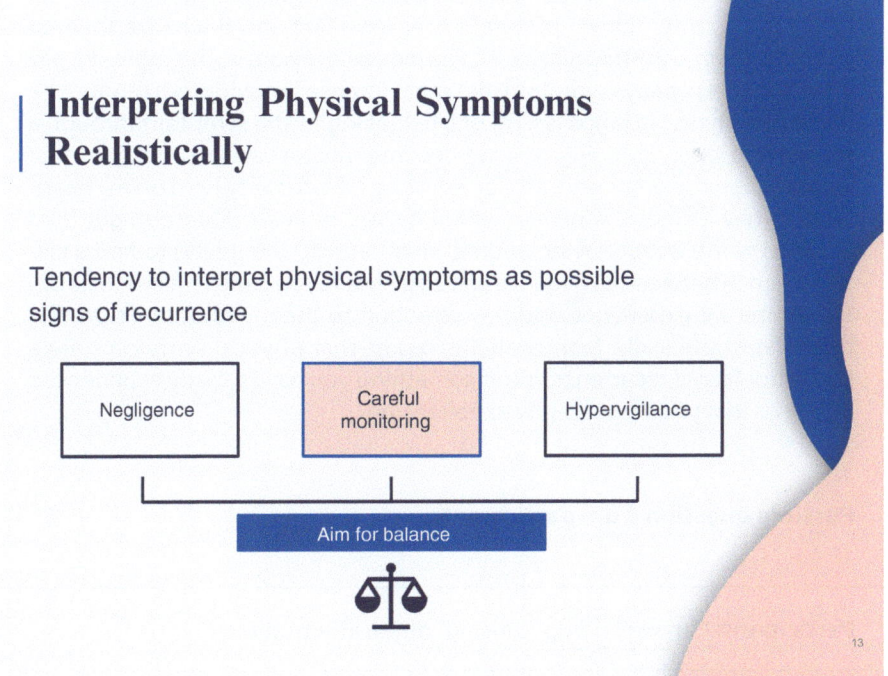

Tell participants that this section aims to help them learn how to interpret their physical symptoms more realistically. Explain that after a cancer diagnosis and treatment, patients often still experience physical symptoms. They may be short-term or long-term side effects of treatment or physical symptoms unrelated to cancer that they have had before, but are interpreted differently after experiencing cancer. Whether we have had cancer before or not, it is practically impossible not to experience any physical symptoms at all in a day, be it pain or other sensations like trouble digesting or muscle stiffness, especially as we age. Our body is constantly active: our heart beats, our muscles are constantly solicited, our digestive system is continuously at work, hormones are liberated in our body, our immune system protects us from infections, and so on. Therefore, it is normal to feel all kinds of physical sensations. Anxiety can also cause many physical symptoms (e.g. shortness of breath, headaches), and they too may be interpreted as signs of cancer recurrence.

> **Facilitator:** There are two types of extreme attitudes that people may have towards physical symptoms. On the one hand, there is negligence, which involves not paying attention to their body at all; this is not necessarily a good thing because they could miss signs of a recurrence or another health problem. It can also be an avoidance strategy that aims to keep their mind off of the disease. On the other hand, there is hypervigilance, which is the tendency to pay attention to every physical sensation and dramatize them or interpret them catastrophically. As mentioned previously, the more we pay attention to a physical symptom, the more intense the symptom tends to be perceived. Hypervigilance is kind of like looking at the symptom through a magnifying glass. By doing this, we become more aware of sensations that would otherwise go unnoticed. For example, if I focus very hard on my heartbeat, it may increase. A person with a history of heart disease might then begin to worry about having another heart attack. The goal is to find a certain balance between negligence and hypervigilance, which means to notice symptoms we experience and pay attention to them without interpreting them catastrophically. Many patients report that physical symptoms are a trigger for fear of recurrence. Is this something you have already experienced before or that you are currently experiencing?

Possible question from participants:

> **Participant:** Can we end up "causing" physical sensations?

Facilitator: Yes. Anxiety can cause many different physical sensations (e.g. muscle tension, numbness, breathing difficulties, digestive problems, etc.), which can be interpreted as potential signs of illness. And the more a person focuses their attention on such symptoms and sees them as a potential threat, the more intense these sensations become, which increases anxiety. Our body is like a radio playing in the background: we all constantly feel sensations such as tingling, tightness, and tension without paying too much attention to them. Hypervigilance can lead us to focus excessively on some of these sensations. By doing so, they may be amplified or even create new symptoms due to anxiety.

Next, explain that people who have a high fear of recurrence tend to interpret their physical symptoms as possible signs of recurrence (and therefore tend to be part of the hypervigilance subgroup). But our subjective perception of the nature of each symptom is not always reliable. Therefore, using objective criteria is an effective strategy to interpret symptoms more realistically.

2.6.2 Slide #14: Interpreting Physical Symptoms Realistically (NILP)

Interpreting Physical Symptoms Realistically (NILP)

Objective criteria	Elise
Novelty	Her symptom is not new
Intensity	Her headache is intense
Likelihood	Her latest test results came back normal; it is rather unlikely that her headache is due to brain metastases
Persistence	To monitor

Present the four objective criteria for interpreting physical symptoms realistically. The first letter of each criterion forms an acronym that is easy to memorize: NILP for Novelty, Intensity, Likelihood, and Persistence. At this point, use the example of a symptom given by one of the participants and analyse it with the group using the objective criteria so they can better understand how to use this strategy. You can also refer to Elise's example that was discussed earlier in the session.

- **Novelty:** Explain to participants that the first step is to ask themselves if their symptom is new. For example, Elise used to have headaches regularly before having cancer, so her symptom is not new. If they have had a symptom for a long time, it is not likely to be due to cancer unless it has gotten worse (second criterion). If you can, take the example of a symptom identified by one of the participants to determine if it is new.

- **Intensity:** Another criterion to consider is symptom intensity. Refer again to the example of Elise's headache. Is it a mild headache that could be relieved by taking Tylenol or Advil, or is it a stronger headache? Is it accompanied by other symptoms such as nausea and dizziness? If so, it is best to see a doctor. Also, go back to the examples of symptoms mentioned by participants and ask them about their intensity. For example, are they more intense or frequent than usual? Do they need to take more medication to relieve them?

- **Likelihood:** Next, tell participants that another objective criterion to consider is the likelihood that their symptom is associated with a cancer recurrence. Refer to Elise's example: she had several tests done recently, and they all revealed normal results. So, in this case, the likelihood that her headache is associated with brain metastases is not very high. Another example you could give participants is a person with a very sore back who was gardening the day before. In this case, it is more likely that their pain is due to the previous day's gardening than to a cancer recurrence. If applicable, also use the examples given by participants.

- **Persistence:** The last criterion is symptom persistence. Point out that it is probably one of the most important objective criteria when evaluating physical symptoms. Once again, refer to Elise's case. Is it a headache that subsides after a few hours, or is it persistent? If a symptom is persistent, suggest setting a time limit after which they will see a doctor and have tests done if the symptom is still present ("If I still have this symptom in X days/weeks, I will go see a doctor"). You can also reiterate the notion of balance between negligence and hypervigilance. Finally, emphasize the importance of giving themselves time, tolerating discomfort, and observing how their symptom progresses before deciding whether to see a doctor or not.

2.6 Interpreting Physical Symptoms

Possible question from participants:

> **Participant:** How long should we wait before seeing a doctor?

Facilitator: There is no absolute rule for this. It depends on the symptom. If it is a severe symptom, such as loss of consciousness or paralysis, you should seek immediate medical attention. However, if it is a common symptom of moderate intensity, such as pain, it would be best to wait for a few days or even a few weeks to see how the symptom progresses. In short, you should use the same criteria that you used before you had cancer. At the time, you probably did not rush to the emergency room as soon as a new symptom appeared.

Facilitator: Whether it is pain, dizziness, numbness, or any other symptom, the aim of the exercise is to objectively analyse physical symptoms to determine whether medical attention should be sought immediately or later. When anxiety is high, there is a risk of seeking medical attention regularly for relatively mild issues and ending up being told: "Like I said the last time, this symptom is nothing to worry about." Has this ever happened to you?

Facilitator: Of course, it is important to remain vigilant because doctors will base their opinion on your observation of your symptoms before ordering extra tests. You should remain vigilant without being hypervigilant. In other words, you should pay attention to your symptoms, but not excessively, to avoid becoming anxious about the slightest headache. Do you feel that this method could be helpful to you? Do you have any questions or comments about it? Asking yourselves these questions does not lead to certainty about the nature of your symptoms, but at least, it allows you to take a step back from them.

2.7 Information-Seeking Profiles

Section objectives:

- **Present the two information-seeking profiles often seen in people who have a high fear of recurrence (i.e. those who want to know as little as possible and those who want to know everything in great detail).**
- **Present the consequences associated with each profile.**
- **Emphasize the importance of seeking a non-excessive level of information that allows them to understand their condition and remain comfortable.**

2.7.1 Slide #15: The Importance of Seeking the Right Information

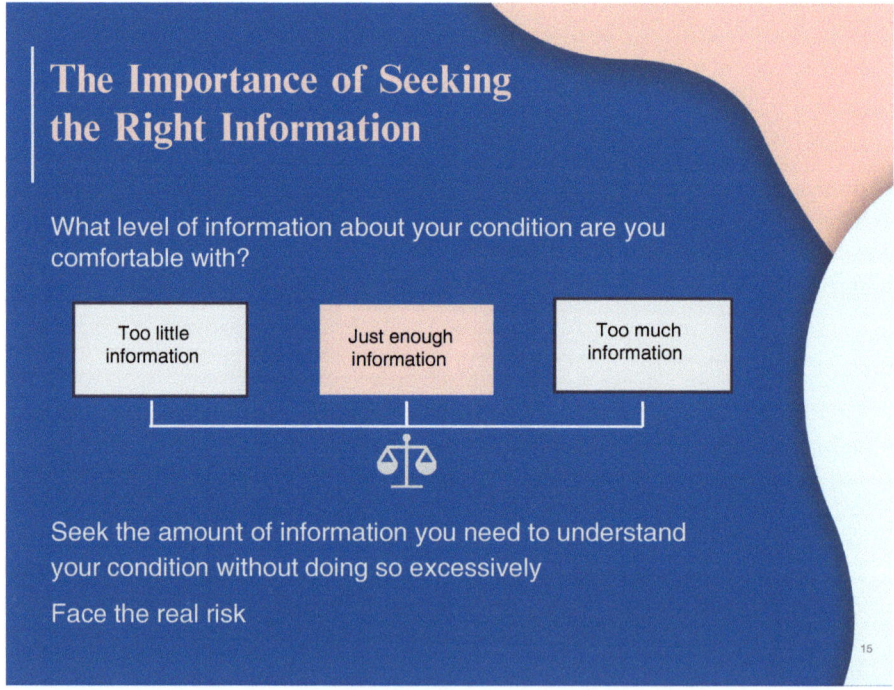

2.7 Information-Seeking Profiles

Facilitator: In the fear of recurrence model, we saw how fear of recurrence is influenced by our level of knowledge about our condition. People's needs may differ regarding the level of information they require about their disease. Some people tend to ask few questions and do not want to seek more information than what is given by health professionals. Conversely, others need to know much more and understand everything. They need to ask more questions and seek information on the Internet (Dr. Google) or books. Does anyone here recognize themselves in one profile or the other, even if their case is not as extreme as those described?

Participant: I don't ask very many questions and I don't read about cancer, but I'm comfortable with that.

Facilitator: Good. Again, the aim here is to find balance. There is no right or wrong way to go about things. However, being in one extreme or the other could be a problem. For instance, wanting to know as little as possible may constitute an avoidance behaviour. This strategy essentially comes down to saying: "Well, the less I know, the less I think about, so the less I worry." Do you think this strategy works?

Participant: No.

Facilitator: Indeed, this strategy rarely works because, most of the time, it creates confusion. For example, just because I don't ask the doctor any questions does not mean that I don't ask myself any questions at all. Without a clear answer from a reliable source, I will eventually find my own answers. If I am anxious, I may find answers that are not entirely reassuring. So, I will end up feeling even more anxious than if I had simply sought the right information. Seeking the right information means facing the actual risk that the disease poses, such as finding out the risk of recurrence of our specific type of cancer. Often, the reality of a situation is not as bad as we feared. We will get to discuss this later.

> **Facilitator:** There are also people who, on the contrary, seek a lot of information. This strategy is generally associated with a need for control. Seeking control over the problems that we can actually control can indeed be a great strategy. However, when we seek excessive control over elements over which we have no real power, this strategy can become problematic. Such is the case for cancer, which is a disease over which we have minimal control. We can also seek information to reassure ourselves. In general, do you find it reassuring to read about cancer on the Internet?

Participant: No. On the contrary, what we find on the Internet is usually a little bit of everything, including some rather dreadful stuff. And the worst part is that we usually fixate on that dreadful information. So, this strategy rarely reduces anxiety.

> **Facilitator:** Exactly! Many patients report that this becomes a new source of concern for them because they discover things they would never have thought of before. In short, you should try to see what level of information you are comfortable with and find a certain balance that will keep you away from the extremes that are generally associated with less effective strategies (avoidance, control and reassurance seeking). In other words, we suggest that you seek the amount of information you need to understand your condition without doing so excessively. Also, remember that when you face the risks you are worried about, you will probably end up finding them much less concerning than you initially thought.

Also, tell participants that they may prefer to avoid asking their doctor certain questions because they do not want to know the answer and do not feel that such information would be helpful. In some cases, this may indeed be preferable. However, it is important to tell them that if they constantly have a specific question on their mind which causes them anxiety, it would probably be best to ask it and face the answer. Knowing what we are up against is preferable to lack of knowledge because the latter leaves room for all kinds of more or less likely scenarios.

2.8 Being Well Informed

Section objectives:

- **Identify with participants the reliable sources of information to which they can refer.**
- **Help participants properly prepare for their medical appointments.**

2.8.1 Slide #16: Being Well Informed

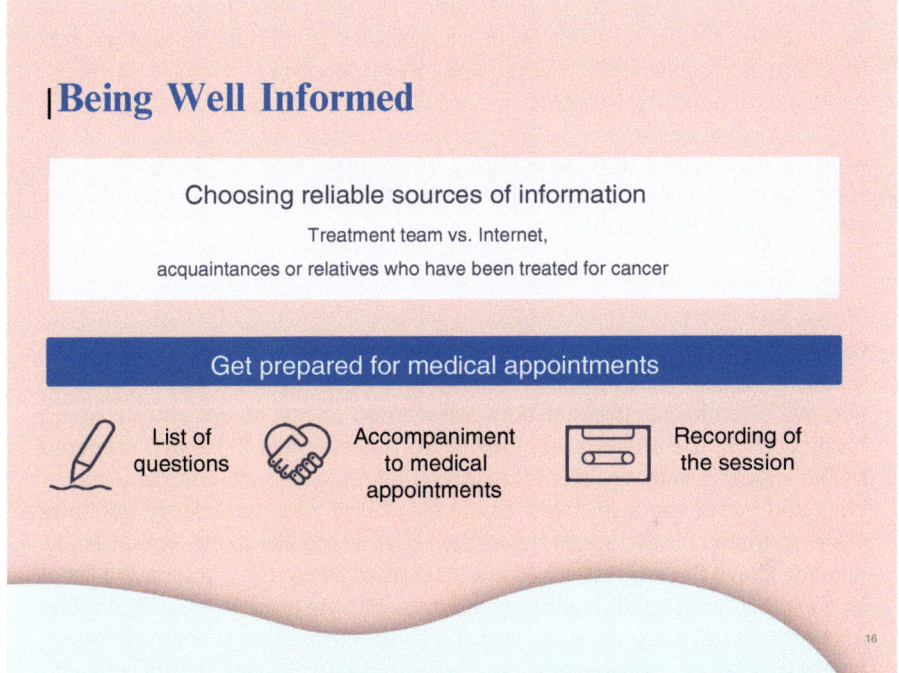

Ask participants if they know which are the best information sources on cancer. Obviously, the most reliable sources are their doctor when accessible and their treatment team, especially nurses. As for the Internet, remind them to be careful because some websites are not very reliable and can even contain all kinds of false information. They can trust some websites, such as that of official cancer organizations, to find reliable information based on the latest research data. However, even on reliable websites, it can be hard to find specific information on their specific type of cancer. Also, warn them about searching for information with vague terms (e.g. headache and cancer), which may lead to results that further increase their anxiety. Remind them that cancer is an overly complex disease and that each condition has its own characteristics. Therefore, they may read something and think it concerns them while this may not be the case, thus leading to confusion and anxiety. In short, recommend that they consult their treatment team first when they have questions or need information on their condition.

> **Facilitator:** Friends and acquaintances can be another problem. You have probably already been told the following: "My neighbour had the same kind of cancer as you, and she was cured after she did…," "So-and-so told me that chemotherapy is…" Remember that such people do not necessarily have the required medical knowledge and the entire picture of your specific medical condition to be in a position to judge what is good or not for you. In short, this type of information is not reliable. It is best to turn directly to your treatment team first when you have questions.

Afterwards, suggest that participants be well prepared before going to their medical appointments. Tell them that seeing their doctor can be stressful, and it is normal to feel a little rushed.

> **Facilitator:** Often, we feel that time is lacking; we do not want to bother the doctor or cause any delay in their schedule. Also, during the medical consultation, we often forget the questions we wanted to ask, so we end up going home without the answers we needed. So, it is essential to be well prepared before meeting with health professionals. Take the time to write your questions down in advance and refer to this list during your medical consultation. Mention that you have specific questions you would like to ask. For example: "Doctor, I have three questions to ask you today." Of course, if you have a list of 15 questions, you probably will not have enough time to ask them all. Therefore, it is best to do a light sorting of them and choose those that seem most important to you. But at the end of the day, you are entitled to a satisfactory consultation during which you receive the information you need. After all, it is their job. Do not be afraid to ask for clarification either, because health professionals do not always realize that their medical jargon is hard to understand.

Next, tell participants that studies reveal that patients forget approximately 50% of the information they are given during medical consultations (Kessels, 2003; Visser et al., 2017). Therefore, a significant proportion of the information discussed is immediately forgotten, mainly because of the anxiety caused by the medical consultation (McClement & Hack, 1999; Rieger et al., 2018). To overcome this problem, suggest that participants attend their medical appointments with another person who could act as a "secretary" by taking notes. This way, they would be able to concentrate more easily and listen more carefully to their doctor. Also, having another person present with them during medical follow-ups could help them validate their interpretation of the information given by the doctor (two heads are better than one!).

Also, mention the possibility of recording medical consultations with a cell phone or another device to avoid missing any information. This way, they could listen to the recording with a clear head after their appointment to improve their understanding of the information they were given during the consultation. Plus, healthcare professionals are generally better communicators when they know they are being recorded. Studies show that audio recordings of medical consultations in oncology are beneficial for most patients, especially regarding knowledge, the sense of being well informed, memorization of information, decision making, and anxiety and depression levels (Rieger et al., 2018). **However, it is crucial to ask for permission before recording the consultation.** A good strategy to help healthcare professionals see this request as acceptable is to specify that you simply want to better memorize and understand the information given during the consultation.

Before moving on to the next section, ask participants if they have any questions or comments about what was just discussed. To stimulate the discussion, you can also ask them if they usually manage to obtain the information they seek during their medical consultations.

2.9   Interpreting Probabilities and Statistics

Section objectives:

- **Help participants understand that their actual prognosis is not necessarily proportional to their level of anxiety about cancer recurrence.**
- **Using examples, explain the following concepts to participants:**
  - Cancer recurrence risk
  - 5-year net survival rate
  - Reduction of recurrence risk based on the proposed treatment
- **Put into perspective the importance of statistics and insist on the importance of realistic optimism.**
- **Help participants understand that statistics constantly change and that current numbers do not necessarily represent today's reality.**

2.9.1 Slide #17: Interpreting Probabilities

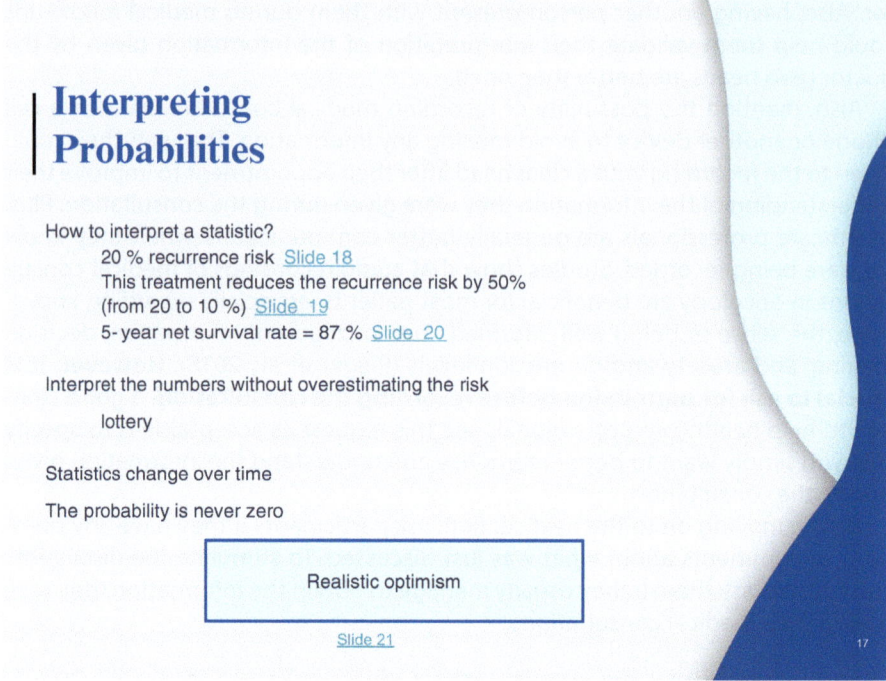

To begin the last segment on realistic interpretation, ask participants about their experiences with probabilities and statistics regarding their disease. Ask them if they have ever asked their doctor these types of questions or if they have ever been told about statistics during medical appointments.

Afterwards, tell participants that it is normal to find it hard to interpret statistics realistically, such as their recurrence risk. It can also be helpful to tell them that the actual statistic is often not proportional to the anxiety they may feel. For example, a person who has a 10% recurrence risk could be 100% anxious about the possibility of a cancer recurrence. Continue by asking them what they think a 20% recurrence risk means.

Explain the following to participants:

> **Facilitator:** Let's look at this question as objectively as possible: a 20% recurrence risk means that in a group of 100 people with cancer with similar characteristics, 20 people will develop a recurrence, and 80 will not. Here is a figure that illustrates this concept.

2.9 Interpreting Probabilities and Statistics

2.9.2 Slide #18: Interpreting Probabilities

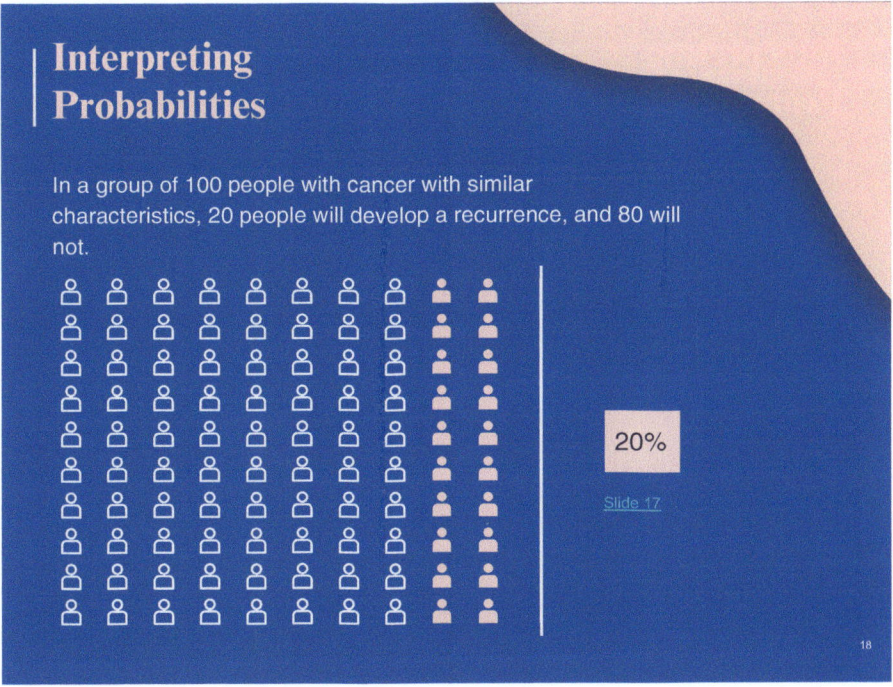

Facilitator: For some people, 20% may seem like a small risk and therefore be very reassuring information, while for others, 20% may seem like a lot because it is still one in five people. In short, the interpretation of recurrence risk can vary a lot from one person to another, but remember that it remains an interpretation that may not be an accurate reflection of reality.

2.9.3 Slide #19: Interpreting Probabilities

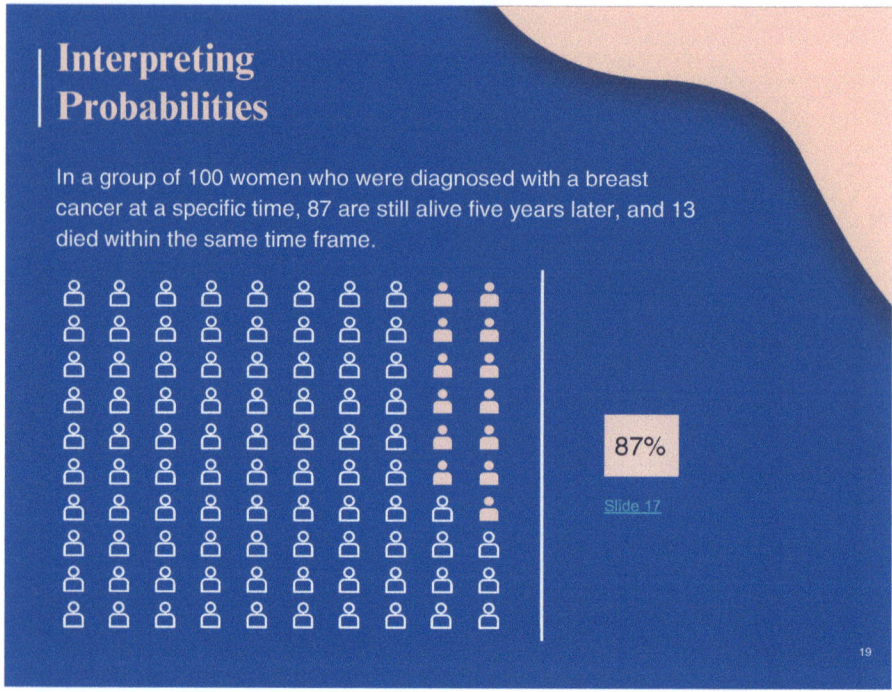

Facilitator: Another cancer-related statistic is the 5-year net survival rate. Has anyone here ever heard about it? Net survival is the probability of surviving cancer in the absence of other causes of death. In short, it is the percentage of people who will survive their cancer. For example, let's say the 5-year net survival for breast cancer is 87%. This means that 87% of women who were diagnosed with breast cancer at a specific time are still alive five years later, and 13% died of their cancer within the same time frame. Note that this statistic improves every year because of constant progress in cancer treatment and early detection.

2.9 Interpreting Probabilities and Statistics

2.9.4 Slide #20: Interpreting Probabilities

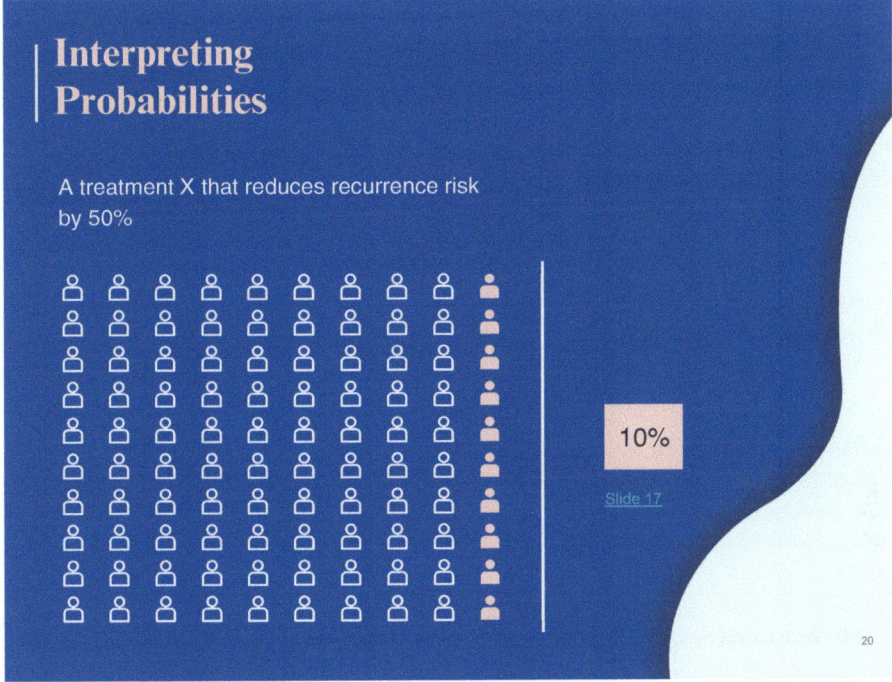

Finally, add that they may have also been told or will be told about the reduction of recurrence risk based on the proposed treatment. Use the example of a treatment that reduces recurrence risk by 50% and explore its meaning with participants.

2.9.5 Slide #17: Interpreting Probabilities (Go Back to a Previous Slide)

Facilitator: The meaning of this statistic depends on your own recurrence risk. Let's take our earlier example of a person with a recurrence risk of 20%. If this person chooses a particular treatment that reduces their recurrence risk by 50%, then their recurrence risk will decrease from 20% to 10%. The number of pink figures would be reduced by half.

Facilitator: If we are taking some time to discuss this subject, it is not to stress the importance of statistics but rather to help you interpret them realistically. Of course, statistics still offer a general idea: recurrence risks of 50% versus 5% are obviously quite different, but statistics and percentages remain very relative. An example we often give to demonstrate the relativity of statistics is lottery. How many of you have already bought a lottery ticket?

Participant: Everyone has probably bought a lottery ticket at least once in their life!

Facilitator: Exactly! So, I suppose that if you bought one, you probably had even just the slightest hope that you would win, right? Otherwise, it kind of would have been like throwing money out the window.

Participant: Yes, my hopes were not that high, but I still had some!

Facilitator: And now, if I told you that there is a new type of lottery where you have a 50% chance of winning a million dollars, would you buy a ticket?

Participant: Yes, for sure!

Facilitator: If we reduced the chances of winning to 20%, would you still want to buy a ticket?

Participant: Yes, the chances are still fairly high.

Facilitator: And if we reduced them to 10%? Or 1%?

Participant: No. The chances of winning would be too low.

Facilitator: The probability of winning the lottery can be as low as one chance out of many millions. Yet, most of you have bought a lottery ticket at least once in your life, if not more. The idea here is that if you once had hope that you could win the lottery with a one in many millions chance and came up with plans for those winnings, then you can also allow yourself to hope that you will not develop a cancer recurrence regardless of your recurrence risk, whether it is 10% or 90%. This way, no matter what statistic is concerned in your case, it is completely justified (and helpful) to remain hopeful that you will be among the subgroup of people who will not develop a recurrence. If you can hope to win the lottery, I think you can also allow yourself to hope that cancer will not come back!

Facilitator: Do you think it is possible to be realistically optimistic with a recurrence risk of 80%?

Participant: Yes, but it would be more difficult…

Facilitator: For sure.

Participant: But you still get to decide how you want to live with that number.

Facilitator: Excellent point! Also, people sometimes defy their prognosis because statistics are approximative.

Participant: Why does the same number seem far worse to us when it concerns disease than when it is related to something more positive like the lottery?

> **Facilitator:** That observation proves that it's not the number as such that influences our reaction, but rather our interpretation of it.

Tell participants that statistics are data that change over time. For example, explain that to determine the 5-year net survival rate, researchers must conduct analyses on patients diagnosed five years earlier to establish whether they survived their cancer within this time interval. Therefore, such statistics are old numbers that may no longer fully apply today. Then, emphasize the fact that the field of oncology is rapidly evolving. Better and more effective treatments are being developed and used that perhaps did not exist when these statistics were first compiled. Conclude by telling them that even if the probability of having a recurrence is never zero, it is still possible to be realistically optimistic and hope to be part of the group of people whose cancer will not come back.

2.10 Cognitive Restructuring Exercise

2.10.1 Slide #21: Exercise to Do at Home

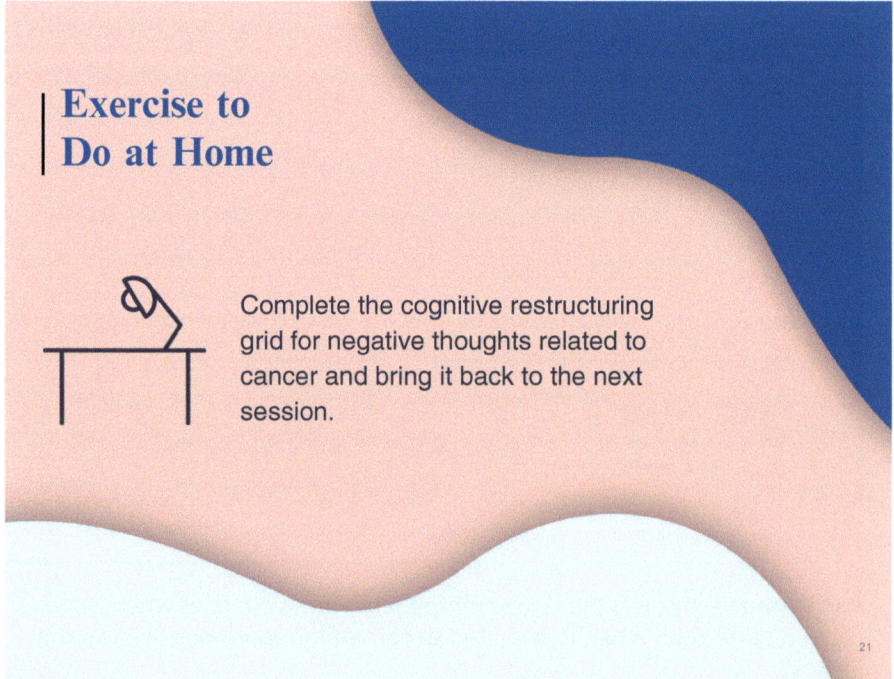

2.10 Cognitive Restructuring Exercise

Explain the cognitive restructuring of negative thoughts exercise that participants are invited to do at home during the week. Give them the exercise worksheet so they can follow along as you explain the exercise. This exercise is an extension of the identification of negative thoughts exercise from the previous week: the worksheet includes the same grid for identifying situations, thoughts, and emotions, but in this particular exercise, additional columns are provided to identify "realistic thoughts" and "emotions" (%). Questions to facilitate cognitive restructuring are also provided on the reverse side of the worksheet. The goal of the exercise is to question the accuracy, validity, and usefulness of negative thoughts with a list of Socratic questions that are meant to challenge a person's initial interpretations. By asking themselves the proposed questions, they may begin to see the situation differently and ultimately change their negative thoughts into more realistic ones. Invite them to write down these elements in the "realistic thoughts" column. Also, tell them that it is usually necessary to come up with several realistic thoughts to counter the powerful effect of negative thoughts.

2.10.2 Slides # 22-23: Cognitive Restructuring Grid and Questionning your Thoughts

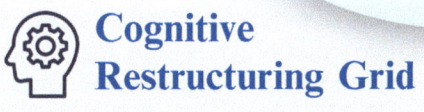

Situation	Negative thoughts	Emotions (%)	Realistic thoughts	Emotions (%)

Beck (1995). Adapted and reproduced with the permission of the author and the publisher.

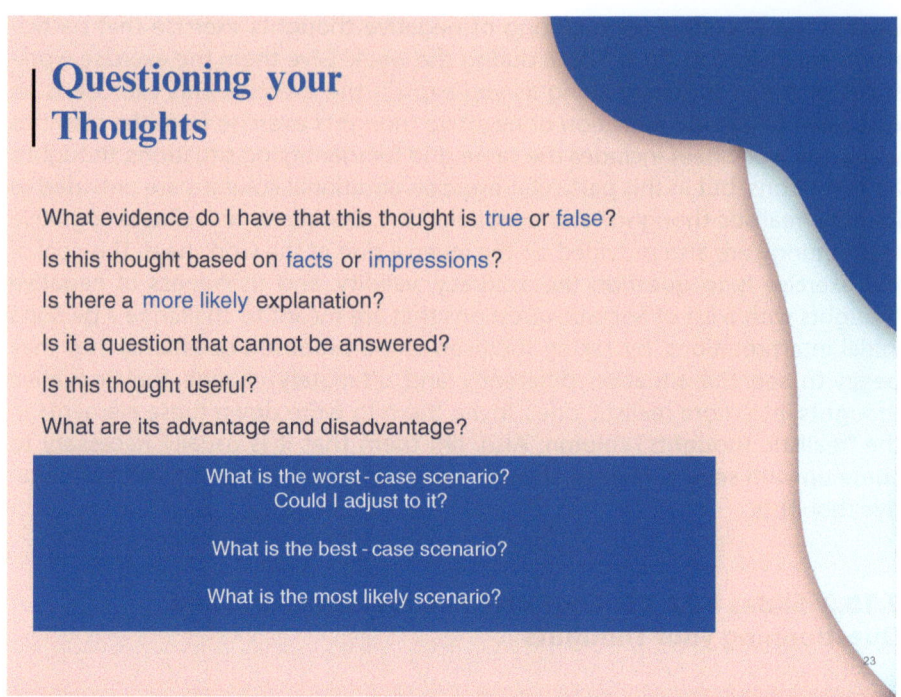

Next, encourage participants to reassess the emotions felt and their intensity once their interpretation of the situation has changed. Specify that a significant decrease in the intensity of their negative emotions is a sign that cognitive restructuring helped them effectively restructure the negative thoughts that were at the root of their emotional state. Likewise, remind them that their emotions may not completely disappear, especially if they are facing a very challenging situation. Tell them that the goal is instead to bring their emotions down to a more tolerable level.

Finally, suggest that they do this exercise for a situation related to cancer or fear of cancer recurrence. However, if such a situation does not occur during the week, tell them that they can also apply cognitive restructuring for other difficult contexts that cause negative emotions, such as a family or work situation.

2.11 Slide #24: End of Session Discussion

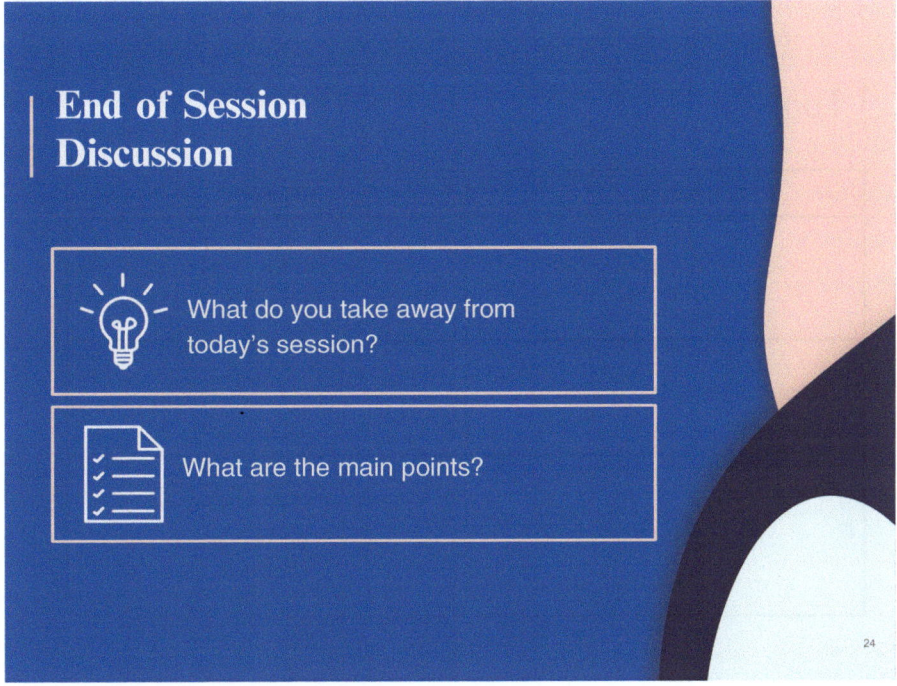

Ask participants what they took away from the session (2 to 4 main points). Also, survey their impressions, appreciation, and comments. Ask them if they have any questions about the content that was presented today.

2.12 Slide #25: Tools in Brief

Tools in Brief

Issues	Solutions
Unpleasant or overwhelming emotions	Cognitive restructuring (grid)
Concerning physical symptoms	Objective criteria (NILP)
Questions/confusion about my medical condition	Make sure I understand well Learn to put things into perspective

Summarize the main strategies discussed during the session for dealing effectively with certain issues related to fear of recurrence:

References

Beck, J. S. (1995). *Cognitive therapy: Basics and beyond*. Guilford Press.

Kessels, R. P. (2003). Patients' memory for medical information. *Journal of the Royal Society of Medicine, 96*(5), 219–222.

McClement, S. E., & Hack, T. F. (1999). Audio-taping the oncology treatment consultation: a literature review. *Patient Education and Counseling, 36*(3), 229–238.

Rieger, K. L., Hack, T. F., Beaver, K., & Schofield, P. (2018). Should consultation recording use be a practice standard? A systematic review of the effectiveness and implementation of consultation recordings. *Psycho-Oncology, 27*(4), 1121–1128.

Visser, L. N., Tollenaar, M. S., de Haes, H. C., & Smets, E. M. (2017). The value of physicians' affect-oriented communication for patients' recall of information. *Patient Education and Counseling, 100*(11), 2116–2120.

Session No. 3

Structure of Session No. 3

Section title	Learning objectives	Page
Session agenda	• Present the topics that will be discussed during the session.	106
Review of the previous session	• Review the highlights of the previous session (questioning negative thoughts, realistic interpretation of physical symptoms and statistics, choosing the right sources of information).	107
Review of last week's exercise	• Invite participants to share their experience. • Remind them of the importance of doing the exercises in writing.	107
Intolerance of uncertainty	• Define intolerance of uncertainty and describe its link with fear of cancer recurrence. • Present the behaviours most frequently associated with intolerance of uncertainty and their consequences on fear of cancer recurrence. • Emphasize the importance of increasing their tolerance of uncertainty and give them a few examples of exposure to uncertainty.	110
Erroneous beliefs about worry	• Explore the various beliefs that participants may hold concerning the usefulness or impact of worrying. • Explain that these beliefs are erroneous and that they may help maintain anxiety.	117
Behavioural avoidance	• Define behavioural avoidance and present its effects on anxiety in the short and long terms. • Explain the concepts of avoidance, behavioural exposure, and habituation with an example. • Present and explain the rules of behavioural exposure (gradual, repeated, and prolonged). • Ask participants about the cancer-related situations they tend to avoid and discuss the impacts of avoidance.	122

Supplementary Information: The online version contains supplementary material available at [https://doi.org/10.1007/978-3-031-07187-4_3].

© The Author(s), under exclusive license to Springer Nature Switzerland AG 2022
J. Savard et al., *Treating Fear of Cancer Recurrence with Group Cognitive-Behavioural Therapy: A Step-by-Step Guide*,
https://doi.org/10.1007/978-3-031-07187-4_3

Section title	Learning objectives	Page
Behavioural exposure exercise	• Suggest an exposure exercise to do at home.	132
End of session discussion	• Ask participants what they took away from the session. • Answer questions and summarize key concepts as needed.	136

3.1 Session Agenda

3.1.1 Slide #3: Session No. 3

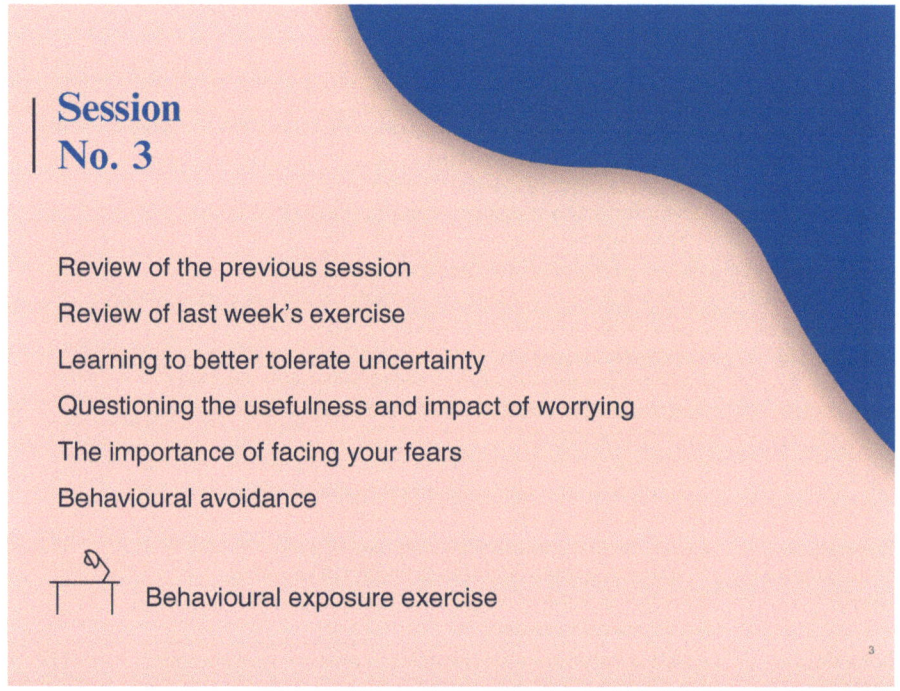

First, present the agenda for the session to participants:
- **Review of the previous session**
- **Review of last week's exercise**
- **Learning to better tolerate uncertainty**
- **Questioning the usefulness and impact of worrying**
- **The importance of facing your thoughts**
- **Behavioural avoidance**
- **Behavioural exposure exercise**

3.2 Review of the Previous Session

Before delving into the content of this session, ask participants if they have any comments, questions, or thoughts that they would like to share about the previous session. Ask them what the highlights of the last session were. Remind them that cognitive restructuring was presented as a strategy to help them change their negative thoughts into more realistic ones. Notions such as realistic interpretation of physical symptoms, statistics, and probabilities were also discussed, and two extreme information-seeking profiles were presented.

3.3 Review of Last Week's Exercise

3.3.1 Slide #4: A Look Back on Cognitive Restructuring

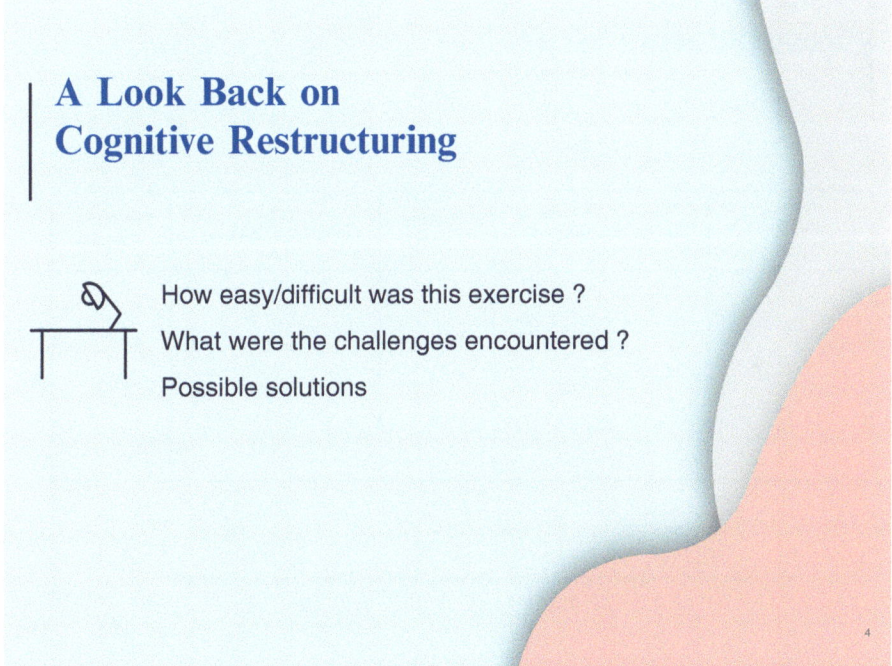

Next, review the exercise that was suggested in the previous session. With the aid of the provided cognitive restructuring grid, the goal of this exercise was to help participants change their negative thoughts. First, they had to identify their negative thoughts. For example, what thoughts crossed their mind when they felt more anxious, worried, or depressed, whether about cancer or not? Second, they had to try to step back from those thoughts by asking themselves various questions (Socratic questioning process). A list of key questions was provided to help them throughout this process. Be sure to specify that it is normal if some of the questions seemed less relevant to them, depending on the situation they experienced and the type of thoughts they had. The goal was simply to help them challenge their negative thoughts from different angles. Then, participants had to come up with more realistic alternative thoughts and evaluate whether such work on their thoughts influenced the nature and intensity of the emotions they felt. Invite them to share their experience with this exercise.

3.3.2 Slide #5: Cognitive Restructuring Grid

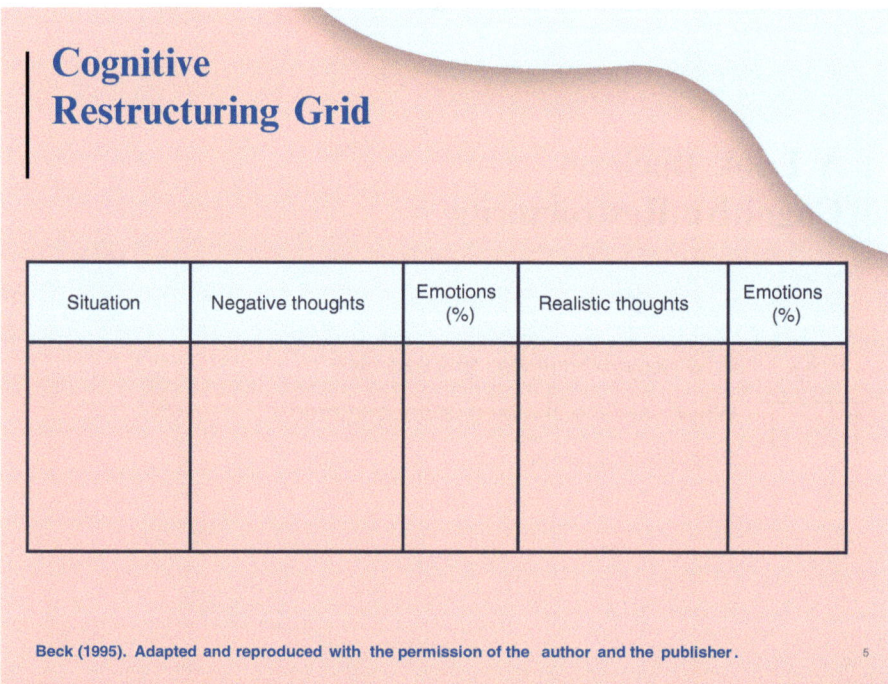

When a participant shares their experience with the group, you can take the opportunity to ask the other participants to come up with other realistic thoughts. You can also invite participants to see you during the break if they have any questions and do not feel comfortable asking them in front of the group or if they want personalized feedback regarding their situation.

3.3.3 Slide #6: Questioning Your Thoughts

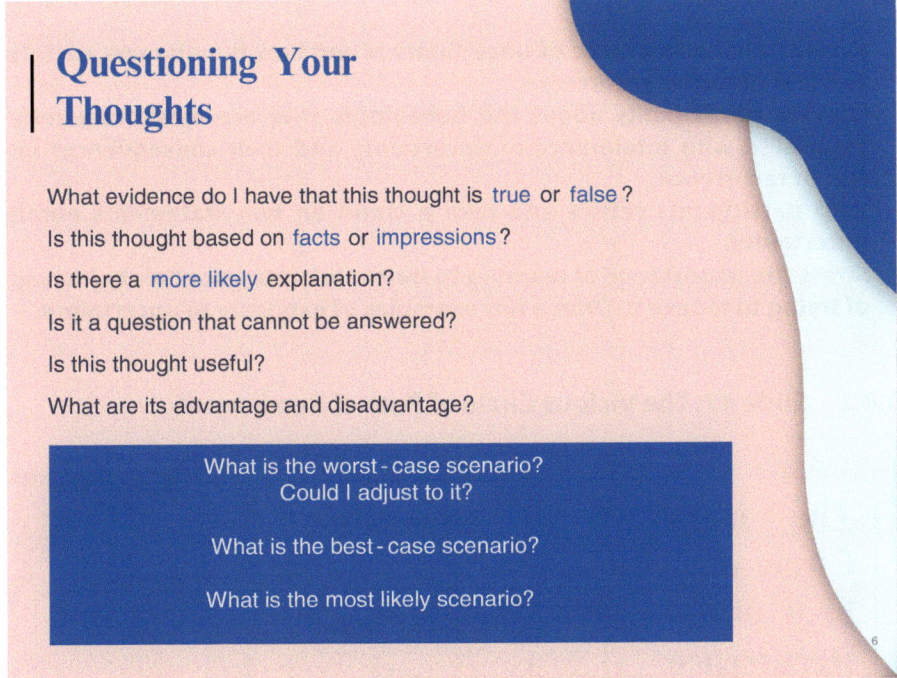

If relevant, take the time to revisit the key cognitive restructuring questions to conclude the review of last week's exercise, with particular emphasis on the question "What is the worst that could happen, and could I adjust to it?"

Remind participants of the importance of doing the exercises in writing. Specify that by writing down their negative and realistic thoughts, it will be easier for them to master this new ability, and they will be able to apply it more quickly when negative thoughts surface. By repeating this exercise, realistic thoughts will eventually come to mind more frequently and spontaneously. Also, remind them that if their knowledge remains at a theoretical level, that is, if they do not apply these new strategies in their life, their effects may be limited. If necessary, remind them of the bike analogy (i.e. the more we practice, the more skilful we become) or the hockey team analogy (i.e. psychotherapy involves teamwork).

3.4 Intolerance of Uncertainty

Section objectives:

- Explain what intolerance of uncertainty is and how it maintains anxiety and fear of cancer recurrence.
- Educate participants about the behaviours that are most frequently associated with intolerance of uncertainty and their consequences on fear of recurrence.
- Help participants reflect and take a stand on two statements about uncertainty.
- Stress the importance of learning to better tolerate uncertainty instead of trying to reduce it. Offer a few examples of exposure to uncertainty.

3.4.1 Slide #7: The Vicious Circle of Fear of Recurrence

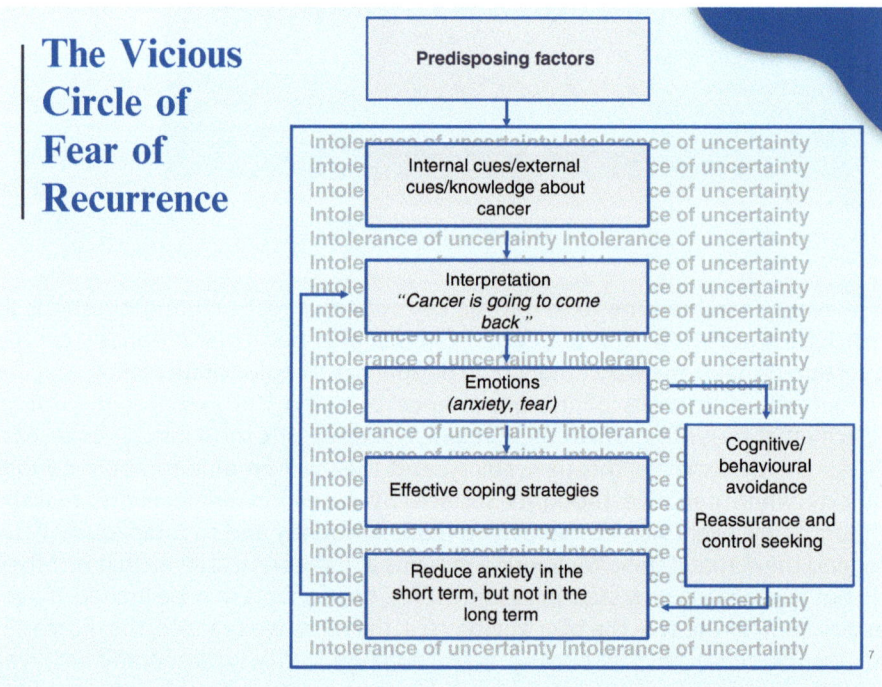

At this point, present the concept of intolerance of uncertainty to participants. Then, present the fear of cancer recurrence model again. Show them that intolerance of uncertainty is illustrated in the background of the model. Explain that this concept was developed in studies on anxiety disorders in particular. These studies have shown that the level of tolerance towards undeterminable

3.4 Intolerance of Uncertainty

outcomes (i.e. uncertainties) varies significantly from one person to another. This means that some people are more intolerant of uncertainty than others. However, specify that once they have become aware of their intolerance of uncertainty, some actions can be taken to reduce it. This point will be discussed in the next few minutes.

3.4.2 Slide #8: Intolerance of Uncertainty

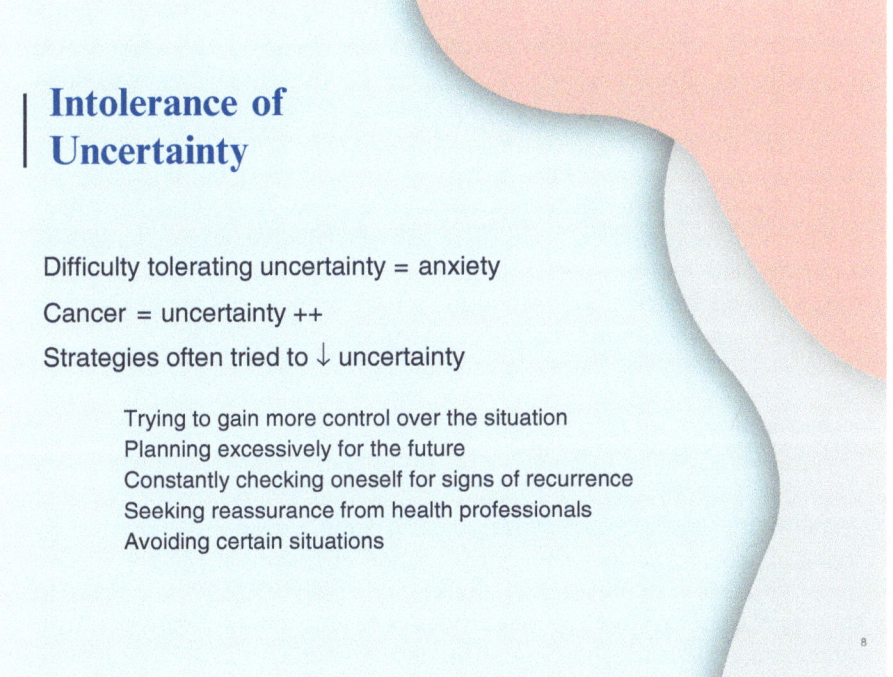

Facilitator: Like a person with a food allergy who reacts strongly when exposed to even the smallest quantity of a specific food, a person who is intolerant of uncertainty (or "allergic" to uncertainty) will react more strongly than others when faced with uncertainty. It has been shown that people who are less tolerant of not knowing what will happen in the future, so of uncertainty, experience more anxiety when faced with uncertain situations. In reality, we all face uncertain situations on a regular basis. Uncertainty is a part of life, so when a person is intolerant of uncertainty, many situations may trigger their anxiety. Uncertainty may be associated with difficult life experiences, such as illness, but also from positive experiences. For example, moving to a new city for a new job is a situation that involves a great deal of uncertainty, even if it is a positive event: "Will I find a suitable house for my family? Will I like my new job? Will I manage to create a new social network? Will the children like their new school and find new friends?" A person who is intolerant of uncertainty or "allergic" to it will have more trouble dealing with such situations.

Facilitator: Cancer is a disease that involves a lot of uncertainty. Right from the beginning of the diagnostic tests, the person is plunged into uncertainty: "Is it cancer? Is it serious? What kind of treatment will I need? How will I respond to it? Will I experience side effects? Will I be cured?" Then, the ultimate question that eventually arises is: "Is it going to come back?" Here, patients may face a great deal of uncertainty because no matter what prognosis they were given, nobody can guarantee that the disease will never come back. If your doctor had told you that your risk of recurrence is 0%, you would not be here today. The uncertainty inherent to the disease and the difficulty you may have dealing with it led you to experience fear of recurrence and to take part in this group. Indeed, fear of cancer recurrence may be stronger and more difficult to manage in people who are more uncomfortable with uncertainty.

Facilitator: So, what do people who are uncomfortable with uncertainty usually do? Often, they will use various strategies to increase their level of certainty that the events they fear will not occur. How do they do this? By trying to gain more control over the situation. For example, people who are uncomfortable with uncertainty often tend to plan things. If we go back to the example of moving to a new city, people who are intolerant of uncertainty and experience this type of situation may spend a lot of time planning this event. They may travel to the new city many months before the move to visit neighbourhoods and schools for their children and map out a specific step-by-step plan for everything. They may even plan solutions to problems that do not exist yet: "If this happens, I will do that." In short, they tend to plan excessively in an effort to gain more control over the situation.

At this point, ask participants if they think that trying to gain more control over what will happen in the future is an effective strategy. Invite them to share their opinions on the subject and ask them if they tend to apply this kind of strategy in their life, and if so, if they find it helpful.

Participant: Yes, sometimes. At work, for instance. I find it helps me to be more organized and efficient.

3.4 Intolerance of Uncertainty

Facilitator: Indeed, in some situations such as at work, the abilities to plan, control, and organize can be assets, qualities that help improve our efficiency. Do you think that planning is an effective strategy in the context of cancer?

Participant: To a certain extent, yes. You have to be responsible, and this requires some level of planning, like for appointments and treatment. To follow medical recommendations, too.

Facilitator: Yes, that is true! But do you think that planning and seeking control are helpful when it comes to the possibility of developing a cancer recurrence?

Participant: No. We don't have total control over cancer, and it's impossible to plan everything.

Facilitator: Exactly. Unfortunately, we don't have total control over cancer. Of course, we can change our lifestyle habits to lower our recurrence risk, but cancer remains a largely uncontrollable condition. Even if we adopt better lifestyle habits, the risk will never be zero. It's not useful to try to gain control over cancer because it's mainly an uncontrollable condition. The same goes for planning what to do if cancer comes back. We cannot plan ahead for everything because the possibilities are endless. When will it happen? How serious will the situation be? Who will be there to help me? Planning ahead for everything is an impossible task. By trying to do so, you might end up planning for events that never occur. What a waste of energy that would be! Planning is a strategy that can indeed be effective in some cases, like in situations we can control. It helps us manage our anxiety about a future that makes us feel insecure, therefore reducing our uncertainty. Since we don't have total control over the possibility that cancer might come back, other strategies should be considered.

Participant: What kind of strategies?

> **Facilitator:** First, you could work on increasing your tolerance of uncertainty! Since you cannot completely eliminate uncertainty, the most effective solution is to accept that life is filled with uncertainty and learn to tolerate the fact that you cannot plan or control everything.

Next, explain that some people may try to gain control over cancer by checking themselves often for signs of recurrence (i.e. self-exams) and being hypervigilant to symptoms to ensure that they could quickly take action if they noticed something abnormal. Also, tell them that people who are less tolerant of uncertainty also tend to seek reassurance, especially from health professionals. Give them the example of a patient who calls their doctor often, asks the nurses many questions, or conducts Internet searches frequently in an attempt to reassure themselves about their condition. This point will be discussed during the next session.

Finally, tell participants that avoidance is another strategy that aims to counter uncertainty. Explain that not thinking about what worries them may give them the impression that what they fear will not happen. However, be sure to specify that this strategy is only effective in the short term. Avoidance will be discussed in more detail later in the session.

3.4.3 Slide #9: What Do You Think of the Following Statements?

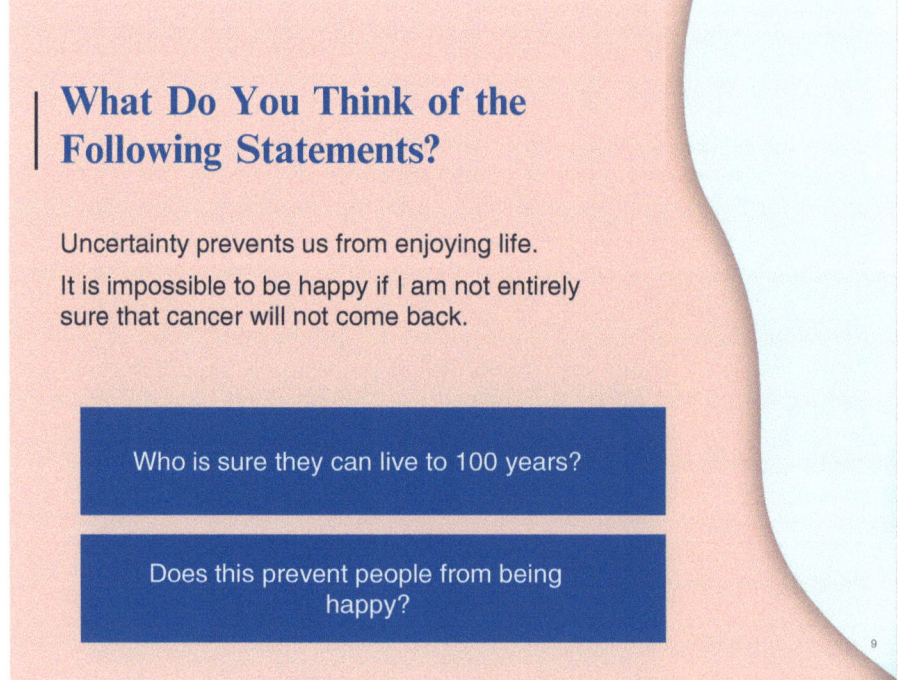

3.4 Intolerance of Uncertainty

At this point, invite participants to reflect on their position towards uncertainty by saying the following:

> **Facilitator:** Now that we have established that uncertainty is inevitable when living with cancer, I would like you to consider the following statements: (1) "Uncertainty prevents us from enjoying life", (2) "It is impossible to be happy if I am not entirely sure that cancer will not come back." What do you think of these two statements? Do you agree or disagree with them?

> **Participant:** I disagree.

> **Facilitator:** Interesting! What makes it possible to be happy despite not knowing whether you will live a long life or whether cancer will come back?

> **Participant:** Enjoying life in the here and now.

> **Facilitator:** Exactly. Enjoying life in the present.

> **Participant:** In the end, lack of certainty in life does not keep us from living.

> **Facilitator:** Absolutely. The only thing we know for sure is that we are all going to die someday. And even if nobody knows whether they will live a long life, this does not prevent us from being happy, having plans in the more or less long term, and enjoying life here and now. We will come back to this point next week. However, we often see that people who had cancer tend to feel that uncertainty is a more significant part of their life because of the risk of cancer coming back. This is not entirely false. However, they did not know whether they would live a long life before their cancer diagnosis either. It is still possible to continue to live fully in the present without worrying too much about any dramatic events that could occur in the future and how they could be managed. Also, uncertainty is not necessarily always negative: the future also has pleasant events in store for us. Think about all the wonderful things that unexpectedly took place in your life. And there are probably many more to come!

3.4.4 Slide #10: Learning to Tolerate Uncertainty

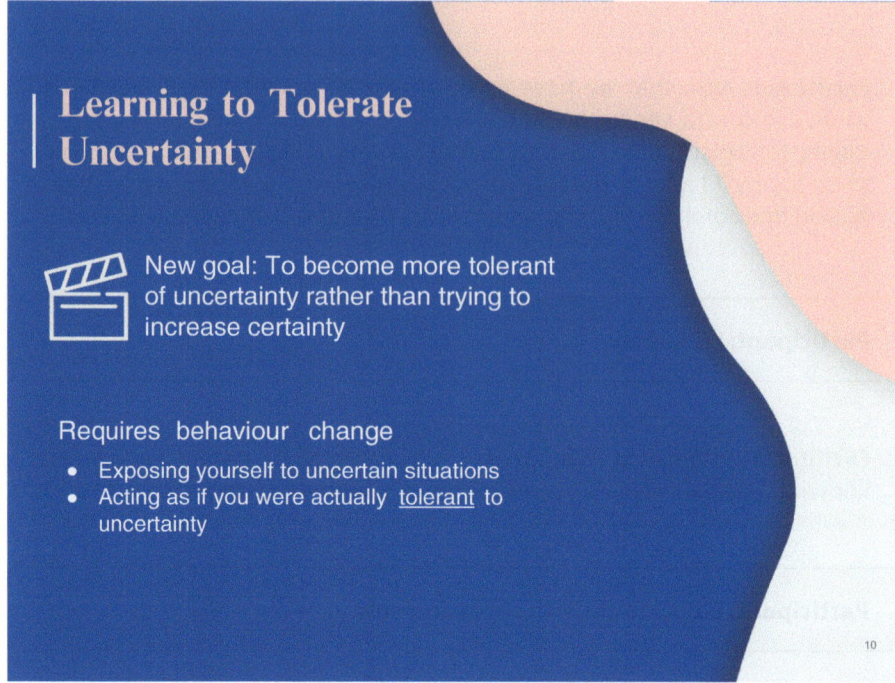

Facilitator: In short, the goal is to become more tolerant of uncertainty. Of course, few people are comfortable with the idea of cancer, but that is not the question we are concerned with here. Some people are naturally more at ease when facing uncertain or unknown situations. For example, some people feel comfortable with the idea of taking a trip without knowing their exact destination or having made reservations for lodging: "We'll see when we get there." Conversely, some people would be unable to tolerate being in such a situation and need to plan everything. The difference between these two types of people rests on the concept of tolerance of uncertainty. A way to increase your tolerance of uncertainty is through behavioural exposure, that is, by putting yourselves into uncertain situations without overplanning. For example, you could go on a trip without a specific plan, lower your weekly menu planning, make fewer lists of things to do, and so on. In other words, the idea is to face situations that make you feel uncomfortable so you can practice becoming more tolerant of uncertainty. Another way to increase tolerance of uncertainty is to act as if you were actually tolerant of uncertainty and tell yourselves: "We will see. I trust myself. I will find a solution when the time comes." The popular expression "I will cross that bridge when I come to it" can be quite helpful in this case.

3.5 Erroneous Beliefs about Worry

Section objectives:

- **Lead participants to reflect on their perception of the usefulness and impact of worrying.**
- **Define what worrying is with participants.**
- **State the various beliefs that participants may hold about the usefulness and impact of worrying and explore whether participants believe any of the following:**
  - Worrying can help us solve problems.
  - Worrying about an event before it occurs can help us avoid experiencing negative emotions (e.g. the emotional reaction after being diagnosed with cancer).
  - Worrying can influence the course of events, either by increasing probabilities (e.g. having an accident or a heart attack) or reducing them (e.g. preventing cancer recurrence).
- **Ask them how they would feel about doing a behavioural experiment (or reality test): would they be comfortable doing one or not? The answer to this question can be a good clue as to whether they hold these kinds of beliefs.**
- **Explain that beliefs about the usefulness of worrying are all erroneous and help maintain anxiety.**

3.5.1 Slide #11: The Usefulness and Impact of Worrying

The Usefulness and Impact of Worrying

1. Worrying can help us solve problems
    "If I worry enough, I will eventually find a solution"

2. Worrying about an event before it occurs can help us avoid experiencing negative emotions
    "If I expect the worst, I will be less disappointed"

3. Worrying can influence the course of the events
    Worrying can make negative events more likely to occur
    "I must not think about that", "I knock on wood"

    Worrying can make negative events less likely to occur
    "If I tell myself that I am cured and let my guard down, cancer will come back"

False beliefs about worries

Next, present the section on the usefulness of worrying. Explain that anxious people often believe that worrying is useful and can influence the course of events.

Facilitator: One of the goals of our program is to help you worry less. I would like to explore the following question with you: Do you feel that worrying can be useful in certain circumstances?

Participant: Yes.

Facilitator: In what kinds of situations?

Participant: In situations that concern our children because sometimes worrying can help us prevent unfortunate events from happening. For example, if I am worried that my child could be kidnapped, I will tell them that they must act in a certain way if something happens. I would also tell them not to talk to strangers.

Facilitator: So, worrying can help us find solutions and prevent unfortunate events from occurring, right?

Participant: Yes.

Facilitator: Okay. Does anyone believe that worrying about something ahead of time can help us better solve problems?

Participant: When our children are concerned, yes, but we should not worry too much either.

3.5 Erroneous Beliefs about Worry

> **Facilitator:** Indeed. But what does it actually mean to worry? Worrying is imagining a more or less likely negative outcome to a situation. Do we really have to worry, that is, to imagine a pessimistic scenario that causes anxiety in order to solve a problem or prevent an event from occurring? If we use your example, is it possible to be aware of kidnapping risks and give your children practical advice to prevent such an event without having to worry about it? Of course, it is! Also, if you worry a lot and make up all kinds of catastrophic scenarios in your head, it may negatively affect your ability to solve problems. In short, worrying does not help us solve problems.

Next, ask participants if they have ever thought that worrying about something could help prevent them from experiencing negative emotions, such as disappointment. Encourage them to elaborate on this subject.

Follow up by asking participants if they had expected to be diagnosed with cancer when they saw their doctor at first. Also, ask if anyone was, on the contrary, convinced that they would receive good news (normal test results). Try to get several answers from the group. Then, ask participants if they think that people who expected to be diagnosed with cancer reacted better emotionally than the others at diagnosis. Conclude by telling them that worrying does not protect us from disappointment and that it only increases distress, not to mention that we often worry about things that do not happen.

> **Facilitator:** In this vein, can worrying influence the course of events? Can it make negative events less likely to occur? Conversely, can it make such events more likely to occur and therefore attract misfortune?

Patients rarely admit or realize that they hold these kinds of beliefs, so tell them that people are not always aware that they have these beliefs. Continue by explaining that a good way to find out whether they hold such beliefs and, if so, challenge them is to do a behavioural experiment.

3.5.2 Slide #12: Behavioural Experiment

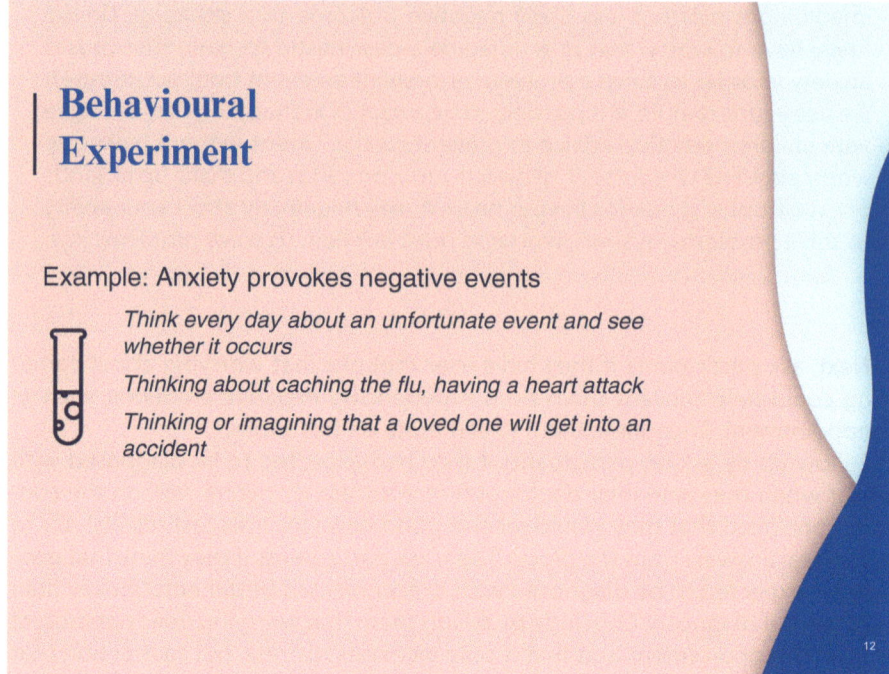

Facilitator: Here is an example of a behavioural experiment or a "reality test" regarding the belief that anxiety provokes negative events. To test whether this belief is true, you could try to think actively about an unfortunate event over the next few days to see whether it occurs. For example, you could think for 20–30 min a day about catching the flu or having a heart attack, or about one of your loved ones getting into an accident, and so on. Would anyone here be uncomfortable doing this kind of exercise?

Participant: (Laughs). Well, I would! I don't want to bring misfortune!

3.5 Erroneous Beliefs about Worry

Facilitator: So, that means that you believe at least a little that anxiety can provoke adverse events, right? This also means that you could benefit from doing this type of experiment. Many patients hold a specific cancer-related belief, that is, that worrying about cancer recurrence will eventually trigger one. This false belief can lead to cognitive avoidance behaviours, which tend to maintain anxiety over time. We will come back to this point later today and next week.

Facilitator: Conversely, some people believe that worrying a lot about something can help prevent the situation from happening, as if remaining alert could protect them from harm. In the context of cancer, this belief may manifest itself in the following way: "I must not tell myself that I am cured, because life could make me regret being so confident and cancer could come back when I least expect it." This belief has adverse effects because if you believe that you need to worry about cancer to prevent it from coming back, it means that you would have to worry all the time. So, you would have no other choice than to remain anxious about it.

3.5.3 Slide #13: Summary

| Summary

- Worrying is not useful and does not influence future events.
- It is essential to challenge these beliefs if you hope to worry less because if you believe that worrying is useful or can influence what happens to you, it will be harder to learn to worry less.
- The future is uncertain: the only control that we have is over our way of adjusting to events when they occur.

> **Facilitator:** The bottom line is that all these beliefs are false: worrying is not useful and does not influence future events. We can conduct behavioural experiments to convince ourselves that such beliefs are erroneous. It is essential to challenge these beliefs if you hope to worry less, both in general and about cancer, because if you believe that worrying is useful or can influence what happens to you, it will be harder to learn to worry less. These beliefs are related to a need for control over the events that we face. But it is just an illusion of control because, as we previously discussed, the future is uncertain and the only control that we have is over our way of adjusting to events when they occur.

At this point, ask participants if they have any questions or comments about what has been said so far.

3.6 Behavioural Avoidance

Section objectives:

- **Define avoidance and explain its effects in the short term (immediately decreases anxiety) and in the long term (maintains and even increases anxiety).**
- **Help participants understand the difference between avoidance and distraction.**
- **Explain the concepts of avoidance, exposure, and habituation using the fear of driving example.**
- **Describe the rules of behavioural exposure.**
- **Help participants reflect on the cancer-related situations that they tend to avoid and give them a few other examples.**
- **Discuss the impact of avoiding these situations with participants.**

3.6 Behavioural Avoidance

3.6.1 Slide #14: The Vicious Circle of Fear of Recurrence

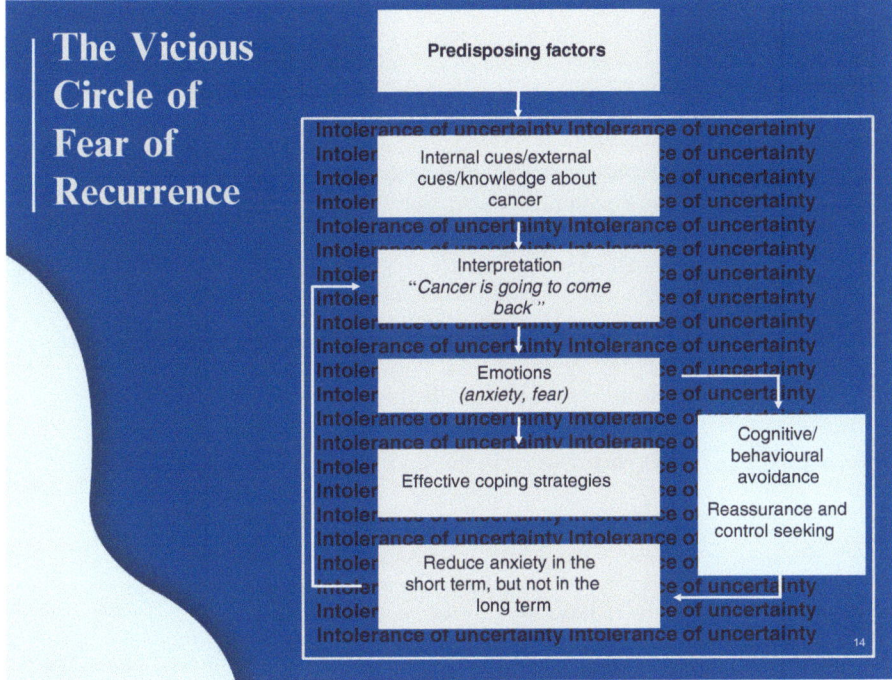

Referring to the fear of cancer recurrence model, tell participants that the last part of the session will focus on behavioural avoidance (cognitive avoidance will be discussed during the next session). Tell them that you will start by offering a general definition of avoidance, after which you will mention its impacts. Then, conclude by telling them about the benefits of behavioural exposure.

3.6.2 Slide #15: Avoidance

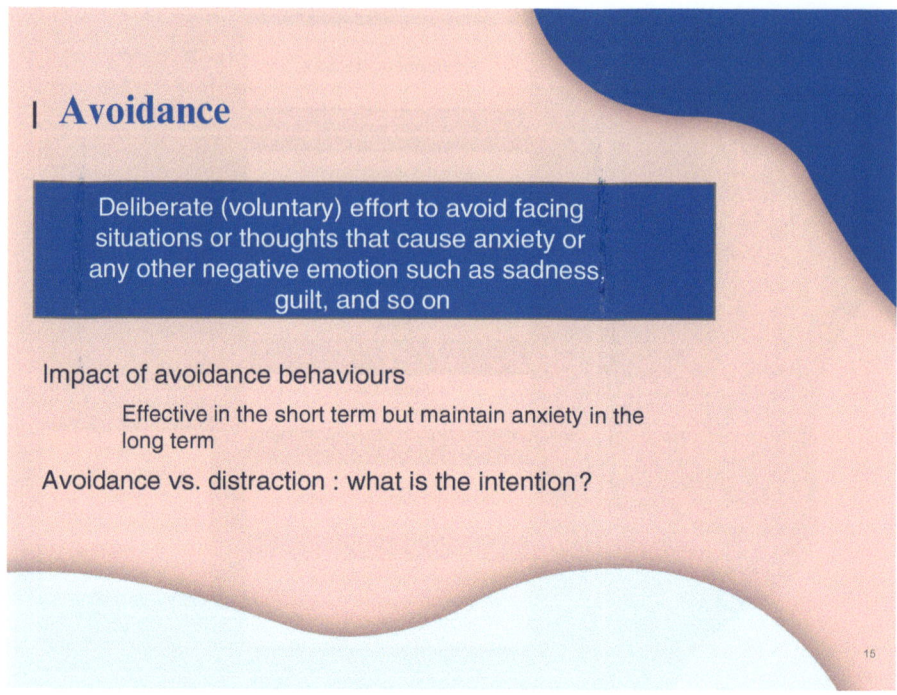

Facilitator: First, we will define avoidance. It is a deliberate (voluntary) effort to avoid facing situations or thoughts that cause anxiety or any other negative emotion such as sadness, guilt, and so on. Avoidance offers instant relief: as soon as we avoid something that we fear or that makes us uncomfortable, we feel better. However, the problem with avoidance is that its effectiveness is only short-lived, and in the long term, it helps maintain and even increase anxiety. Why? Because by practising avoidance, we end up confirming to ourselves that we have escaped a form of danger. So, the next time we face the same situation, we will interpret it as a threat.

3.6 Behavioural Avoidance   125

> **Facilitator:** Here, it is important to note that avoidance should not be confused with distraction. Engaging in pleasant activities or discussions with others about topics other than cancer out of pure pleasure is obviously not the same as doing an activity to avoid thinking about something that frightens us, such as cancer recurrence. To determine whether a behaviour is a form of avoidance, you must ask yourselves about your motives and intentions for doing something. For example, am I doing crossword puzzles because I enjoy this activity or because I do not want to think about cancer? The answer to this question is crucial.

3.6.3 Slide #16: Avoidance and Habituation Curves

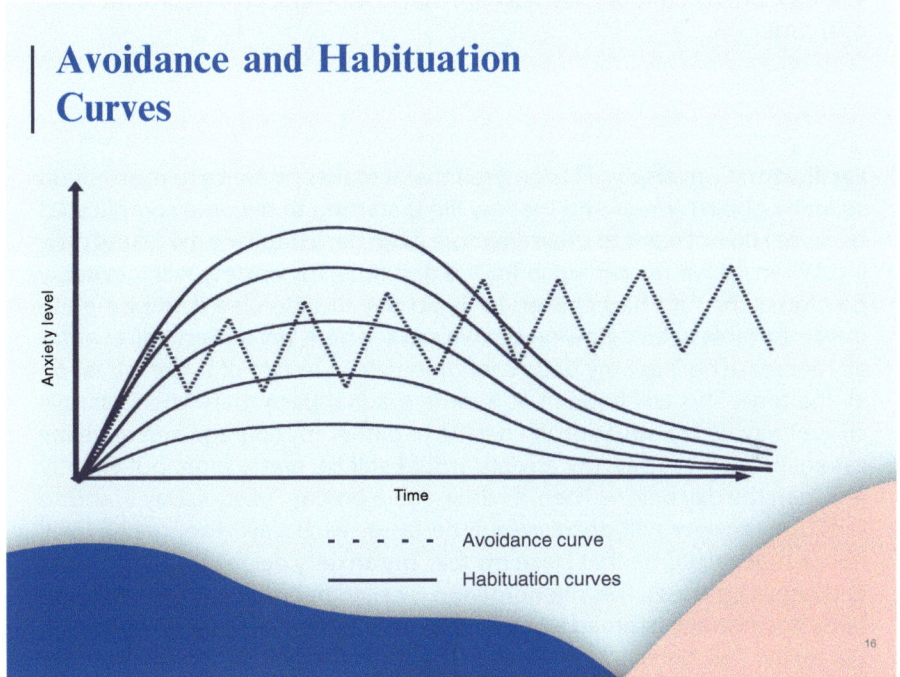

Facilitator: Now, I will show you the avoidance curve, which is the zigzag line in the graph. First, let's use an example unrelated to cancer. Let's imagine that I had a car accident, which was quite a traumatizing experience. Obviously, I would feel very anxious about driving again and would be tempted to avoid this situation as much as possible. But at some point, I will have to go to an appointment or to work. It would be easier to drive my car there, but the idea of driving makes me anxious. If I decide to take the bus, I will avoid having to drive, which will relieve my anxiety. This is an effective solution in the short term. However, the problem with avoidance is that the next time I have a trip to make, my anxiety will be just as high as the first time, if not higher. Then, it will decrease just as fast when I decide to avoid the situation again by taking the bus or simply avoiding going to the scheduled event. In short, I will avoid facing the situation to relieve my anxiety temporarily, which will lead me to believe that avoidance is an effective strategy. On the contrary, we see here that driving anxiety tends to increase over time.

Facilitator: Conversely, if I tell myself that it makes no sense to miss out on so many opportunities and that my life is starting to become complicated because I do not want to drive anymore, I can decide to face my fear of driving. When I drive my car again for the first time, my anxiety will inevitably be higher than if I had chosen to avoid the situation, so it will be quite uncomfortable at first. However, as we can see here, my anxiety will eventually decrease because my body cannot remain in a state of hyperactivation all the time. This will happen at a more gradual pace than when I simply chose to avoid the situation. If I decide to gather my courage and drive my car again the next day, my anxiety would still be pretty high, but slightly less than the day before. Then, if I drive again on Day 3, Day 4, Day 5, and so forth, my anxiety will decrease a little faster each day. Eventually, I will notice that each time that I face my fear, my anxiety decreases a little more and lasts a little less. This phenomenon is called habituation: the brain and body become accustomed to a situation, so they do not react as much to it. But most of all, behavioural exposure helps us realize that the situation we fear is not as dangerous as we thought.

Facilitator: Here, you have probably noticed that the anxiety does not necessarily drop to zero, even after facing the situation repeatedly. Do you know why?

3.6 Behavioural Avoidance

> **Participant:** We know that driving always involves a risk.

Facilitator: Exactly. This is true for situations that generate strong fear, like cancer, so we cannot become completely desensitized to it. The goal of behavioural exposure is not to eliminate anxiety altogether, but rather to reduce it to a point where it becomes less overwhelming and debilitating.

3.6.4 Slide #17: Behavioural Exposure Rules

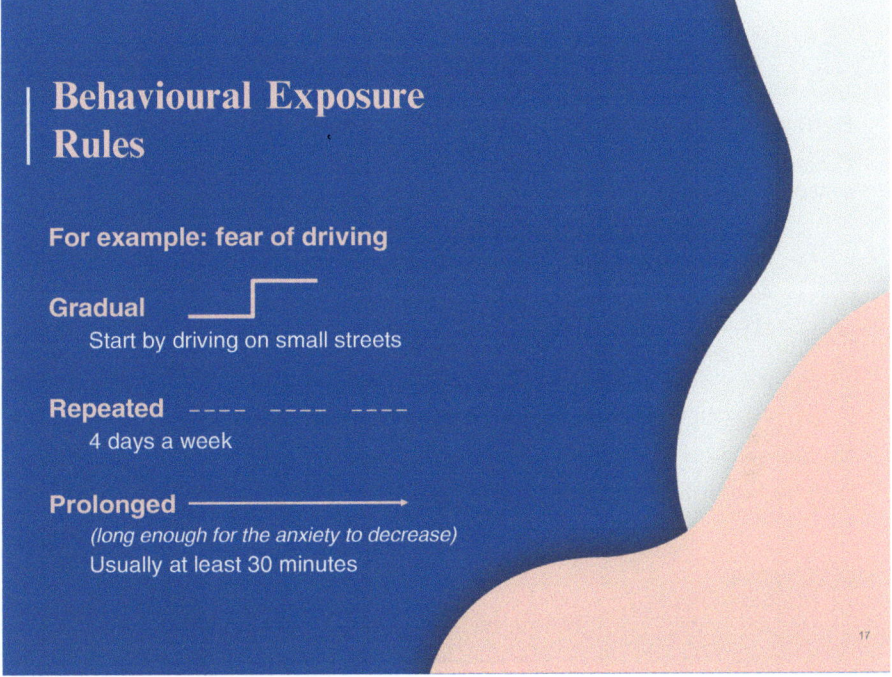

At this point, explain the rules of behavioural exposure to participants. Tell them that ideally, behavioural exposure to the feared object or situation should be done gradually. You can use the driving example. First, the person may start by driving on small streets. Once their anxiety has sufficiently decreased, they will be able to start driving on avenues and boulevards, then on highways. If desired, they can begin the process with someone accompanying them, then go driving alone. Behavioural exposure must also be done frequently, for example, daily. Again, illustrate this rule with the driving example. Suppose a person decides to drive their car on a particular day and only drives it again a month later. In that case, their brain will not remember that it went well the first time and that their anxiety had eventually decreased because too much time has passed between the two exposure sessions. Finally, explain to participants that behavioural exposure must be conducted over a prolonged period. For example, if a person takes their car for a short distance and gets out just a few minutes later, their anxiety will not have time to decrease as seen in the habituation curve. The person will then remain stuck in their negative experience and may not want to start over again. Therefore, each behavioural exposure session must be long enough to allow anxiety to have time to decrease (usually at least 30 min).

3.6.5 Slide #18: Avoidance and Cancer

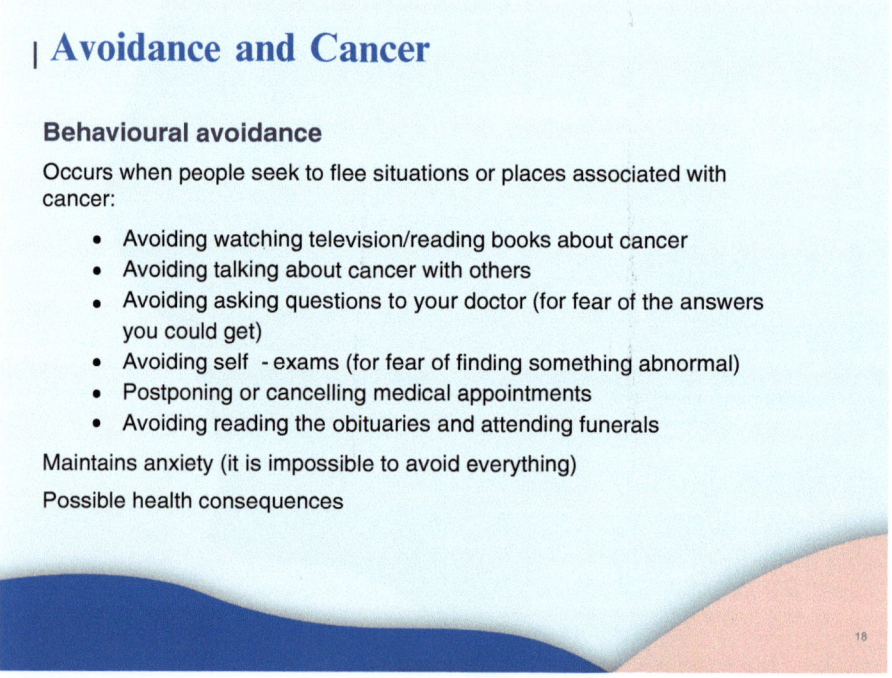

At this point, ask participants to give examples of situations they tend to avoid since experiencing cancer. Here is an example of a discussion with participants:

3.6 Behavioural Avoidance

Facilitator: Are there any situations that you tend to avoid since your cancer diagnosis?

Participant: Yes.

Facilitator: What kinds of situations?

Participant: Well, I don't like to talk about cancer.

Facilitator: So, you avoid conversations on the subject?

Participant: Yes.

Facilitator: Okay. Does anyone else avoid any cancer-related situations?

Participant: I used to visit online forums on cancer, but I can't do that anymore.

Facilitator: Why?

Participant: I don't like it. It seems like it's all just bad news. It doesn't make me feel better at all.

Participant: The same goes for me. I used to be in a Facebook group where I saw plenty of cases of recurrence. I ended up finding it was too much for me, so I left the group.

Facilitator: These are good examples. So, because visiting those websites made you feel anxious about your situation, you decided to stop. At a glance, this would indeed seem to be a form of avoidance. However, as mentioned previously, keep in mind that discussion forums are not the best place to find reliable information on cancer. It is best to consult other more reliable sources.

Possible question from participants

Participant: I'm having trouble with the concept of behavioural exposure. I don't see how reading or watching television shows about cancer or hearing stories about cancer recurrence will help reduce my anxiety. I don't feel like hearing about it, and I don't see what I have to gain from it! Do I really have to do this?

Facilitator: Thank you for bringing up this point! This leads me to specify that avoidance becomes a problem when it demands a lot of effort and prevents us from doing things that are important to us. You may not feel that this is true for you because it is not necessarily a problem in your life.

Participant: Yes, but at some point, isn't it normal not to want to hear about it anymore?

Facilitator: Yes, but as I said earlier, you have to figure out the intention behind your actions. Let's say you don't read cancer articles that you come across. Is it because they stir up anxiety that you have trouble managing or because you're not interested in these articles and are sick of hearing about cancer? If the answer is the former, this is a form of avoidance, and you could benefit from facing your fear instead of avoiding it because avoidance maintains anxiety over time.

3.6 Behavioural Avoidance

Next, do a brief review of behavioural avoidance with the participants by presenting different situations they may tend to avoid. Use both the examples given by participants and those mentioned below.

Here is a list of examples to explore with participants:

- Avoiding asking questions to your doctor for fear of the answers you could get
- Avoiding self-exams for fear of finding something abnormal
- Postponing, delaying, or neglecting medical appointments or check-ups
- Not talking about cancer with others
- Avoiding running into certain people for fear of being asked about your cancer
- Avoiding watching television shows or listening to the radio, reading books or newspaper articles about cancer
- Avoiding reading about your type of cancer (documents given by the medical team, reliable websites)
- Fleeing from hospitals, waiting rooms, blood tests, etc.
- Avoiding reading the obituaries
- Avoiding attending funerals

Next, specify the following:

> **Facilitator:** Cancer is such a widespread disease that it is impossible to avoid everything related to it, even if such avoidance is motivated by a lack of interest or being fed up rather than by anxiety. You can't stop watching television or using the Internet, or completely prevent people from talking to you about cancer. These situations are avoidable, but only to a certain extent.

> **Facilitator:** Finally, some rare forms of avoidance are more serious than others. For example, postponing or cancelling medical appointments can have significant health consequences. Therefore, it is crucial to reduce such avoidance behaviours sooner rather than later.

3.7 Behavioural Exposure Exercise

3.7.1 Slide #19: The Importance of Facing Your Fears

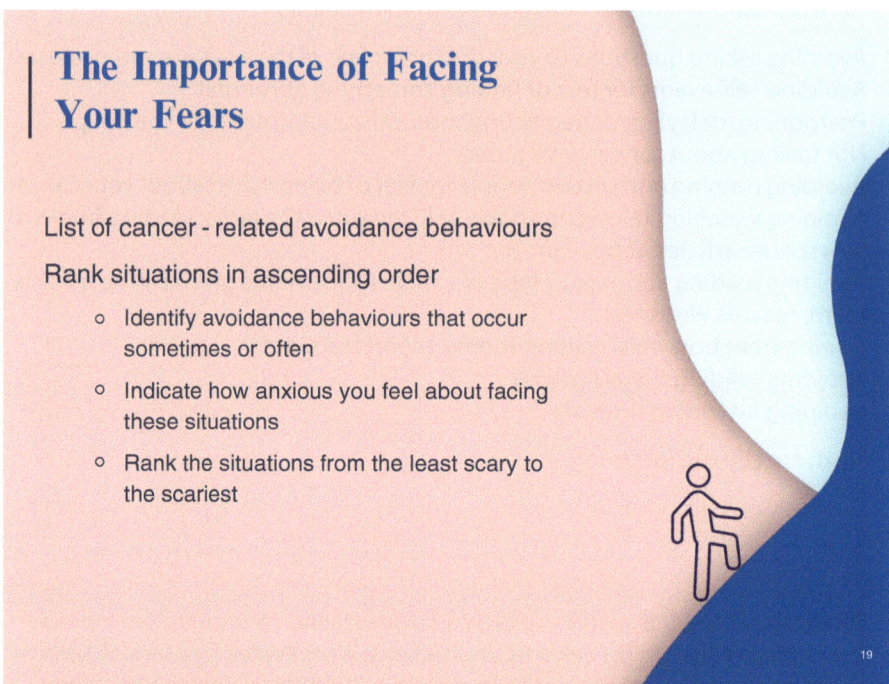

At this point, explain this week's exercise to do at home. Give participants a list of common cancer-related avoidance behaviours that they may adopt to avoid feeling anxious. Ask them to look at the list of situations and indicate how often they avoid each one (i.e. never, sometimes, or often). Next, ask them to note the percentage of anxiety they would feel if they faced each situation they avoid at least "sometimes". Ask them to rank the situations in ascending order, that is, from the situation that makes them the least anxious to the one that makes them the most anxious. Ask them if they have any questions and if the exercise instructions are clear so far.

3.7 Behavioural Exposure Exercise

3.7.2 Slide #20: Exercise to Do at Home

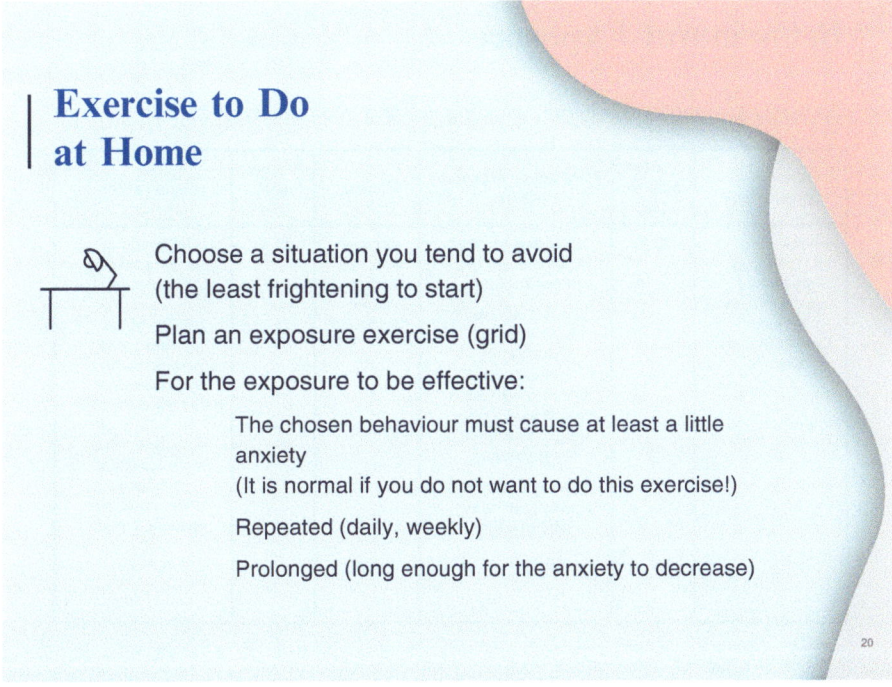

Continue explaining the exercise by asking participants to choose a situation they tend to avoid. They should choose one that is associated with less anxiety to start. However, their chosen behaviour must cause them at least a little anxiety for the exposure exercise to be helpful. Tell them that it is normal if they do not want to do this exercise as it involves confronting a situation that causes them anxiety. Remind them that behavioural exposure must be prolonged (i.e. long enough for the anxiety to decrease) and repeated (e.g. daily).

3.7.3 Slide #21: Behavioural Exposure

Behavioural Exposure

Targeted avoidance behaviour: avoiding reading information on cancer

Behavioural exposure task	Anxiety before (%)	Behavioural exposure actions	Results	Anxiety after (%)	Observations
Reading information on my type of cancer on the Canadian Cancer Society website	70 %	Reading for 30 minutes every day for 7 days Starting with the least stressful sections (e.g., treatment) and finishing with the most stressful ones (e.g., recurrence, metastases) Planning a pleasant activity to do after the session	Anxiety was high at first, then it decreased	30 %	I felt proud of myself for reading this content Some of the content I read answered some of my questions about my condition At the end, I feel more confident because I understand my disease better

Finally, present the following example to participants:

Facilitator: Here is the example of a person who avoids reading about cancer and finally decided to face their fear. We can see how they plan to read information about cancer on the American Cancer Society website, starting with the least anxiety-inducing sections. They intend to read some information on the website for 30 min every day for a week. Afterwards, they plan to reward themselves by doing a pleasant activity. We can also see that their initial anxiety about doing this exercise was at 70%. During the exercise, they tolerated the discomfort they felt, waited for it to decrease, then noted their observations in the grid.

3.7 Behavioural Exposure Exercise

Invite participants to write down the results of their behavioural exposure exercise. For example, they may have found it unpleasant due to high anxiety at first, then felt better afterwards. Ask them to write down their observations and anything positive they got out of the exercise. Like the person in the example, they may feel proud of themselves for having dared to face their fear (e.g. reading information about cancer) or more confident because they understand their disease better.

At this point, issue the following warning:

> **Facilitator:** A small clarification is in order here. In the example we presented, we see how the person's anxiety has considerably decreased. However, if you decide to confront something you are very afraid of, your anxiety may not decrease as much during the first behavioural exposure sessions. In fact, it might even increase. Bear in mind that this is normal. You may have even experienced the same thing with this therapy group. Perhaps you sometimes leave the group with a higher level of anxiety than when you first arrived. However, with practice and repeated exposure to the situation you fear, your anxiety will eventually decrease.

At this point, ask participants if they have any questions or comments about the exercise or avoidance and behavioural exposure in general.

3.8 End of Session Discussion

3.8.1 Slide #22: End of Session Discussion

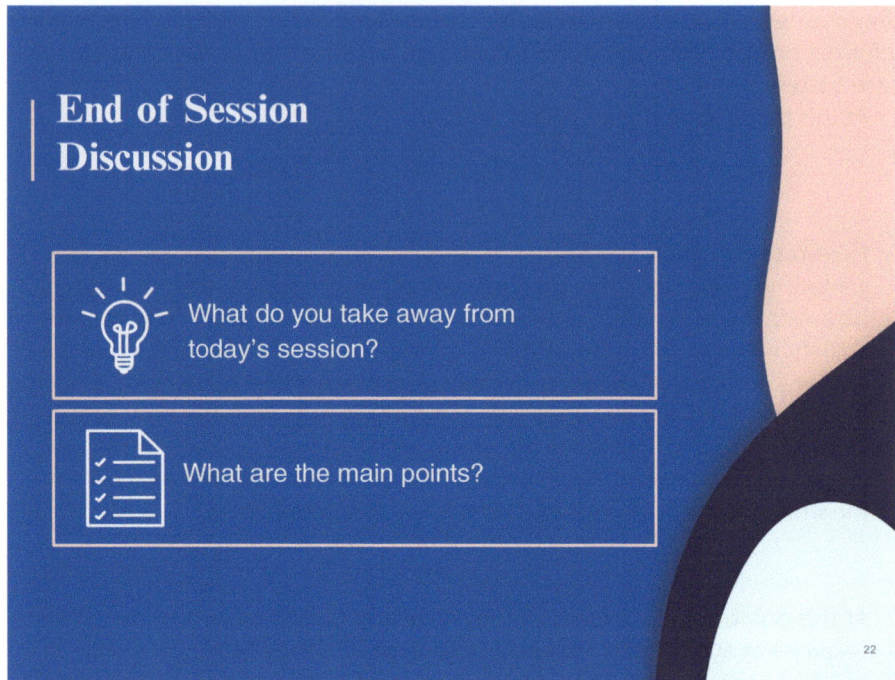

Ask participants what they took away from the session (2 to 4 main points). Survey their impressions, appreciation, and comments. Ask them if they have any questions about the content that was presented today. Remind them that the idea of behavioural exposure is to get them to face situations that cause them anxiety so they may eventually see that their anxiety decreases with exposure to these situations. It is essential to remind them that behavioural exposure will not completely desensitize them to the feared situation, that is, a possible cancer recurrence. However, they will discover their ability to manage their fear better. Remind them that avoidance helps maintain anxiety in the long term. Also, by avoiding situations for fear that they would be too upsetting, they remain convinced that they cannot overcome them. This is an idea that exposure allows to test and disprove. Often, the experience turns out to be much less difficult than initially expected.

3.9 Slide #23: Tools in Brief

Tools In Brief

Issues	Solutions
Intolerance of uncertainty	Exposure to uncertain situations Act as if I were more tolerant "Let go of control"
Belief that worrying is useful	Question my beliefs Do a behavioural experiment
Tendency to avoid situations that make me think about cancer	Plan a behavioural exposure exercise (grid)

Summarize the main strategies discussed during the session for dealing with certain issues related to fear of recurrence effectively:

Session No. 4

Structure of Session No. 4

Section title	Learning objectives	Page
Session agenda	• Present the topics that will be discussed during the session.	141
Review of the previous session	• Review the highlights of the previous session (intolerance of uncertainty, erroneous beliefs about usefulness and impact of worrying, behavioural avoidance).	142
Review of last week's exercise	• Invite participants to share their experience. • If necessary, remind them that behavioural exposure must be frequent and long enough to have a beneficial effect on anxiety.	143
Cognitive avoidance	• Define and explain cognitive avoidance. • Point out that it is normal to use this strategy. • Help participants understand that cognitive avoidance contributes to the vicious circle of fear of cancer recurrence by making thoughts more frequent and overwhelming. • Encourage them to direct their efforts towards strategies that are more beneficial in the long term.	145
Strategies to counter cognitive avoidance	• Present and explain the most effective strategies for dealing with negative thoughts (cognitive restructuring, planned worry time, acceptance and cognitive exposure).	151
Seeking reassurance	• Define and explain reassurance seeking. • Present the clues that allow to distinguish reassurance behaviours that are excessive from those that are adaptive (intention, degree/intensity). • Remind participants that it is impossible to eliminate all doubts and, as such, excessive reassurance seeking is an ineffective strategy to deal with anxiety.	159

Supplementary Information: The online version contains supplementary material available at [https://doi.org/10.1007/978-3-031-07187-4_4].

© The Author(s), under exclusive license to Springer Nature Switzerland AG 2022
J. Savard et al., *Treating Fear of Cancer Recurrence with Group Cognitive-Behavioural Therapy: A Step-by-Step Guide*,
https://doi.org/10.1007/978-3-031-07187-4_4

Section title	Learning objectives	Page
Seeking control	• Present some behaviours that may be adopted to increase the sense of control over the disease (physical exercise, diet, visualization). • Help participants understand the difference between habit changes that aim to improve quality of life versus those made in an attempt to gain control over the disease. • If needed, review the risk factors for cancer recurrence based on currently available research (tobacco, alcohol, obesity, etc.). • Highlight that there is no such thing as an anti-cancer lifestyle, that scientific data are constantly evolving on factors influencing cancer, that it is important to have realistic goals with regards to lifestyle changes, and that pleasure is important in life.	163
What if cancer comes back?	• Reiterate that if a recurrence were to occur, it could progress in many different ways (not always fatal). • Remind participants of the importance of considering all possible scenarios while hoping for the best (realistic optimism).	166
Redefining life goals	• Help participants understand the importance of having life goals (they give them purpose in life). • Explain that it is always possible to have life goals that are adapted to their values and capacities. • Emphasize that the important thing is not necessarily to achieve life goals, but rather to take action to move closer towards what is important to them. • Propose some exercises to help them identify goals that have meaning for them and that are likely to enrich their life.	170
End of session discussion	• Ask participants what they took away from the session. • Answer questions and summarize key concepts if needed.	179
General review of the psychotherapy group	• Ask participants what they took away from the four sessions. • Answer questions and review the key concepts if needed. • Explain that the next step is to put into practice the newly learned strategies in order to try to change certain harmful behaviours or attitudes identified during the sessions.	181

4.1 Session Agenda

4.1.1 Slide #3: Session No. 4

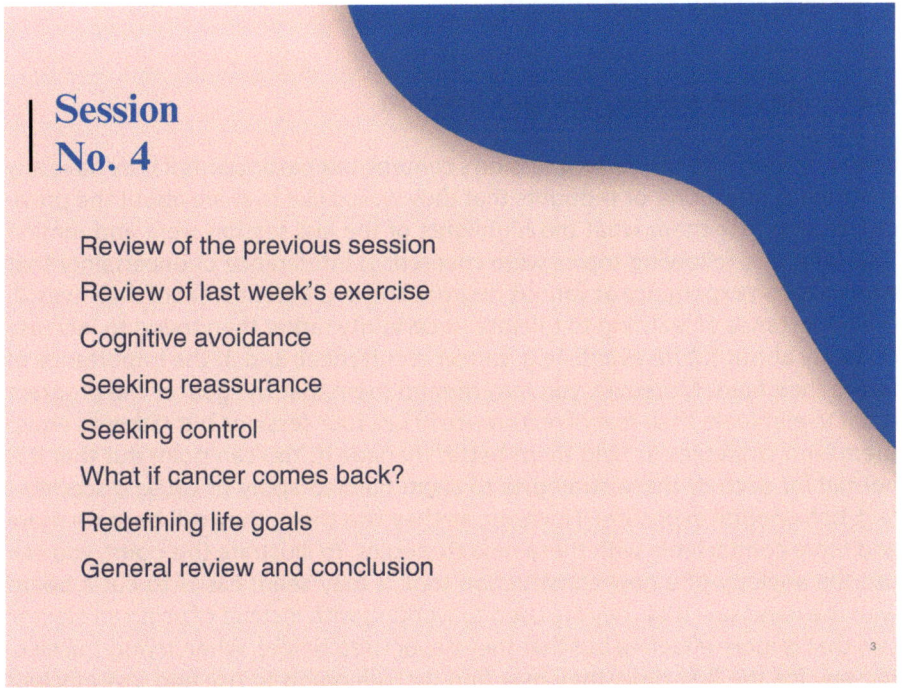

First, present the agenda for the session to participants:
- **Review of the previous session**
- **Review of last week's exercise**
- **Cognitive avoidance**

- **Seeking reassurance**
- **Seeking control**
- **What if cancer comes back?**
- **The importance of life goals**
- **General review and conclusion**

4.2   Review of the Previous Session

Before delving into the current session's content, ask participants if they have any comments, questions, or thoughts that they would like to share about the previous session. Ask them what the highlights of the last session were and remind them that the following topics were covered: 1) intolerance of uncertainty that everyone can experience at various degrees and in different areas of their lives; 2) the importance of learning to tolerate uncertainty rather than trying to increase certainty about future events (e.g. cancer recurrence); and 3) the importance of facing their fears. Moreover, you may remind them that the goal of the program is not to eliminate their fear of recurrence in just four sessions but rather to equip them with strategies to help them better manage it. You can point out that it is normal for each of these strategies to seem hard to apply or cause discomfort (e.g. behavioural exposure). However, as they use them, they will become more and more comfortable with these new strategies. To illustrate this point, you can use the analogy of a new construction tool: It may seem easier to cut a board with the hand saw that they are used to working with instead of using an electric saw that is more effective but that they never used before. When trying the electric saw for the first time, they may find it challenging to use and less efficient than their hand saw. However, in time, they will become able to use it more easily and efficiently.

4.3 Review of Last Week's Exercise

4.3.1 Slide #4: Review of the Behavioural Exposure Exercise

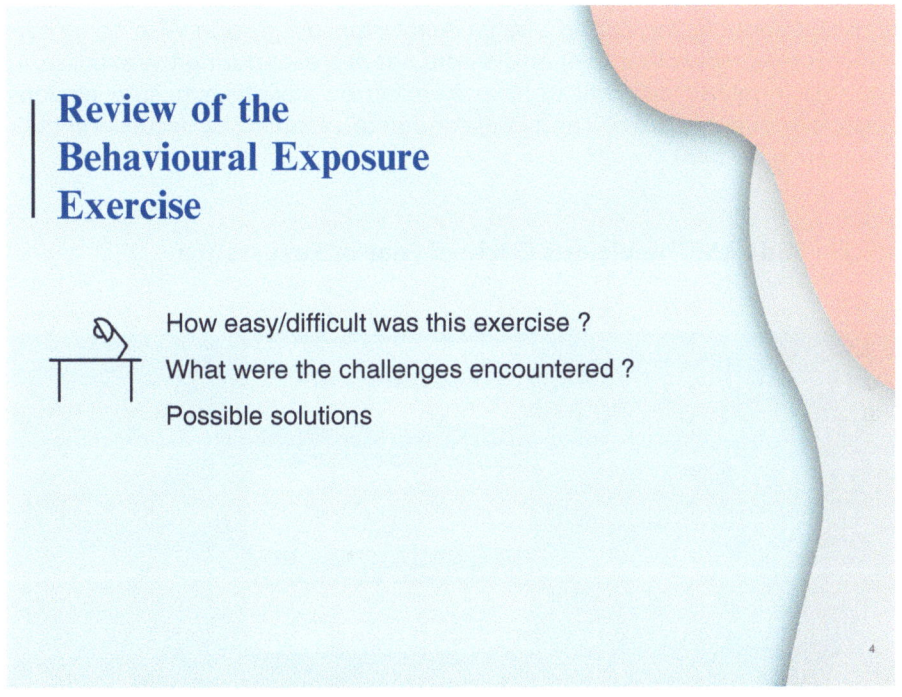

Next, review last week's exercise with participants. If they are comfortable doing so, ask them to share their thoughts and experiences with the behavioural exposure exercise. Ask them if they came across any obstacles during the exercise. Some participants may report that they did not do the exercise because it caused them too much anxiety. If so, you could review the list of situations they tend to avoid and help them identify one that they would feel more confident about facing during a behavioural exposure session. Also, some participants may report that their anxiety did not decrease during the exercise. In that case, remind them that to have an effect on anxiety, exposure sessions must be frequent (e.g. daily) and long enough to experience a decrease in their anxiety (e.g. 30 min).

4.3.2 Slide #5: The Vicious Circle of Fear of Recurrence

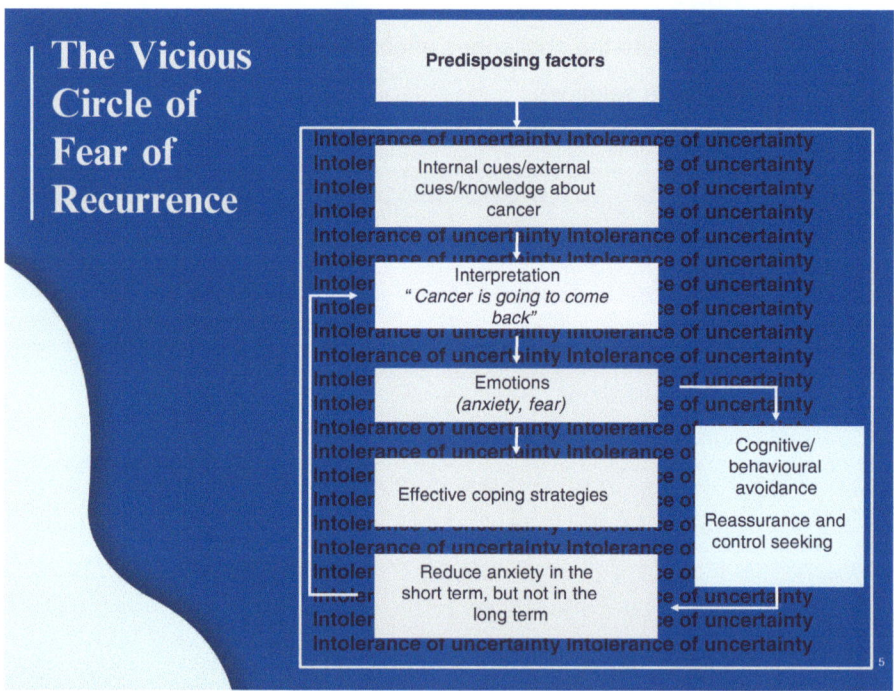

While reintroducing the vicious circle of fear of cancer recurrence, tell participants that the following minutes will be dedicated to cognitive avoidance and seeking reassurance and control.

4.4 Cognitive Avoidance

Section objectives:

- **Help participants understand that avoiding thoughts requires a lot of effort and tends to have the opposite effect of the one desired by increasing our focus on thoughts that we want to avoid.**
- **Define cognitive avoidance and give a few examples.**
- **Explain how cognitive avoidance helps maintain the vicious circle of fear of cancer recurrence by making thoughts more frequent and overwhelming.**
- **Point out that it is normal to use this strategy on a daily basis because of its short-term effectiveness.**
- **Encourage them to direct their efforts towards strategies that are more beneficial in the long term.**

4.4.1 Slide #6: Cognitive Avoidance - The Camel Exercise

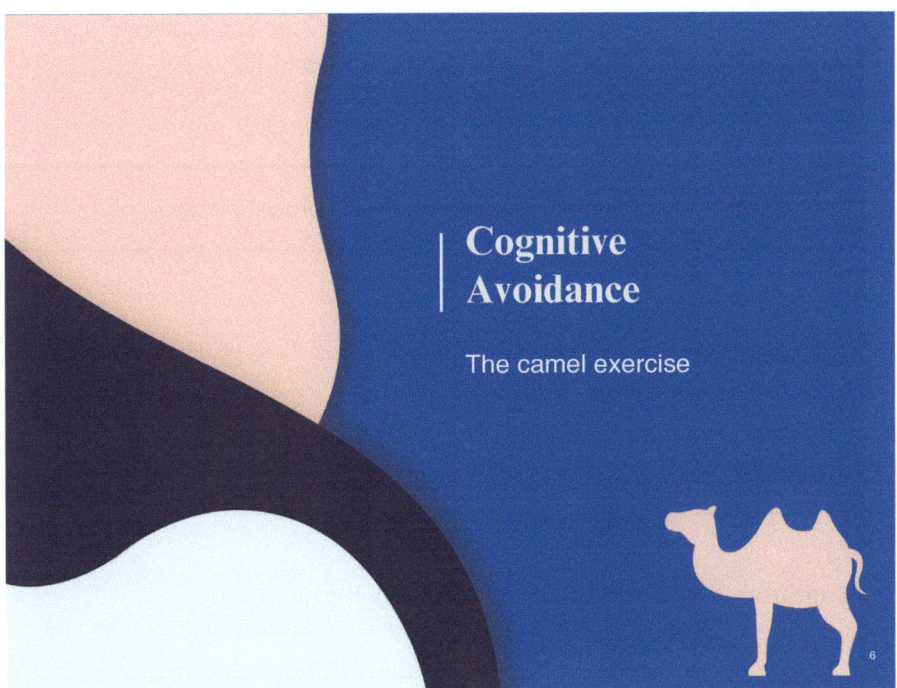

With the participants, do an exercise that demonstrates the effect of cognitive avoidance: the camel exercise.

Exercise: Step 1

> **Facilitator:** For the next minute, I would like you to close your eyes and concentrate very hard on only one thing: thinking about a camel. Don't think about anything other than a camel. Try doing this exercise, and we will talk about it afterwards.

> **Facilitator (after 1 min):** Okay, you may open your eyes now. What did you notice? Were you really able to keep the image of a camel in your mind during the whole exercise?

Participant: Yes, pretty much.

> **Facilitator:** No other thoughts popped into your mind?

Participant: The image did leave my mind, but I brought it back.

> **Facilitator:** Did it require effort to do that?

Participant: Yes, some effort.

> **Facilitator:** Some effort because other thoughts popped up?

Participant: Yes. I had other thoughts.

> **Facilitator:** Did anyone else experience this too?

4.4 Cognitive Avoidance

Participants: Yes!

Exercise: Step 2

Facilitator: For the next minute, I would like you to close your eyes and do the opposite exercise: think about anything you want, except a camel. Each time the camel pops into your mind despite all your efforts, please raise your hand.

Facilitator (after 1 min): Okay, you may open your eyes now. What did you notice during this exercise?

Participant: The camel was there the whole time!

Facilitator: It was there the whole time?

Participant: Yes!

Facilitator: Was this the case for anyone else? Did the camel come back despite all your efforts not to think about it?

Participant: Sometimes it went away, sometimes it came back.

Participant: I thought about a forest and the camel appeared in it!

Facilitator: What you described is very representative of what generally happens. Do you know why the camel popped into your mind even when you made an effort to think about something else?

Participant: Because we were told not to think about it?

Facilitator: Exactly. In short, this exercise demonstrates how hard it is to think about only one thing, as we have seen during the first part of the exercise, but also that it is even more difficult to force ourselves to not think about one thing. Avoiding thoughts requires a great deal of effort. You may have also noticed that forcing yourself to not think about something actually has the opposite effect. Paradoxically, the more we try not to think about something, the more our focus shifts to it. In this case, it shifted to the camel.

Facilitator: Of course, the camel is a pretty harmless thing to think about for most people. However, when unpleasant emotions are attached to an unwanted thought, such as the possibility of cancer coming back, it becomes even more difficult to get rid of it. Trying to not think about something makes us think about it even more.

4.4.2 Slide #7: Cognitive Avoidance

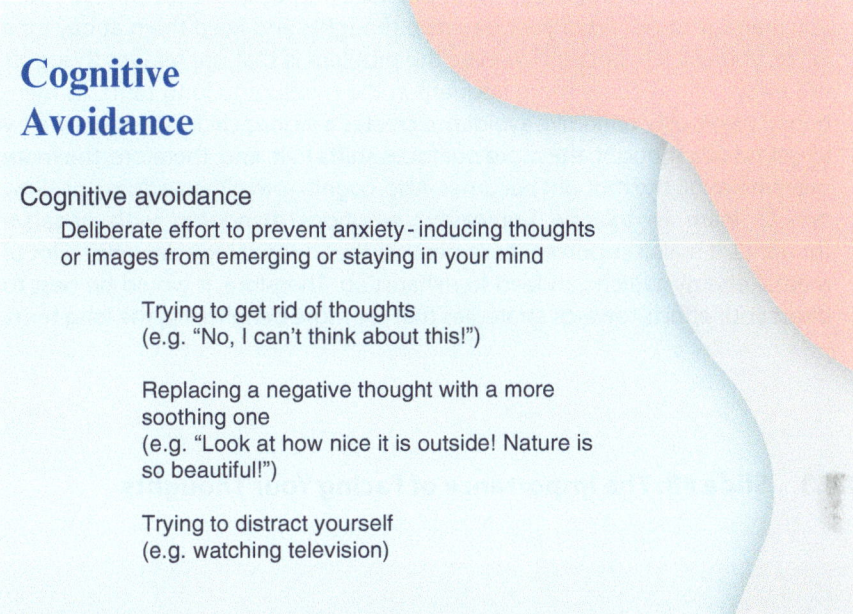

Give participants a more specific definition of cognitive avoidance, or, in simpler terms, thought avoidance. Tell them that it is a deliberate (voluntary) effort to prevent anxiety-inducing thoughts or images from emerging or staying in their mind, such as those related to cancer. Next, give them a few examples of cognitive avoidance: trying to get rid of thoughts ("No, I can't think about this!"), replacing a thought that makes them uncomfortable with a more soothing one ("Look at how nice it is outside! Nature is so beautiful!"), and trying to distract themselves (e.g. watching television).

Facilitator: There is a reason why we practise cognitive avoidance. Like behavioural avoidance, this strategy often provides immediate relief. At first, when you manage to get rid of your negative thoughts and keep them at bay for a while, you will feel better. However, the problem is that unpleasant thoughts will eventually become more frequent in the medium to long term. As mentioned previously, cognitive avoidance creates a vicious circle: The more we try to get rid of a thought, the more our focus shifts to it, and, therefore, the more overwhelming the thought becomes. Also, cognitive avoidance does not allow one to learn to tolerate unpleasant emotions associated with negative thoughts. It is also important to remember that this strategy demands a lot of mental energy, which can lead to exhaustion. Therefore, it would be best to direct your efforts towards strategies that are more beneficial in the long term.

4.4.3 Slide #8: The Importance of Facing Your Thoughts

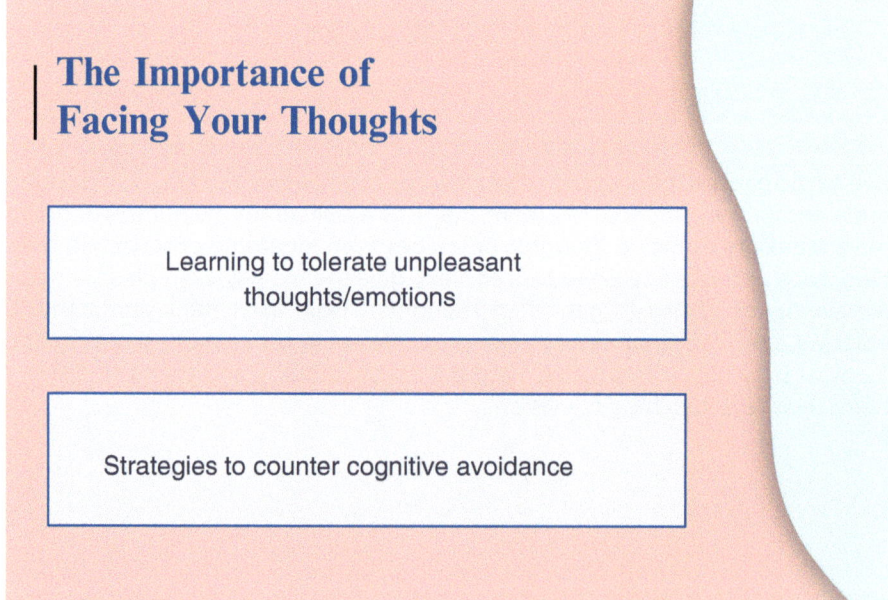

Facilitator: For these reasons, we encourage you to face your unsettling thoughts in order to reduce your anxiety. This involves learning to tolerate catastrophic thoughts and scenarios instead of trying to eliminate or escape them. We are going to present a few strategies to help you learn to better tolerate your negative thoughts.

Possible question from participants

Participant: I don't think about it and I'm fine with that. I don't see why I should force myself to think about it. That would be torture!

Facilitator: I know that it may seem counter-intuitive to do this. If not thinking about cancer or a possible cancer recurrence doesn't demand any effort, then indeed, perhaps these strategies would not be relevant in your case. It is really when it requires an effort not to think about something that it becomes important to face your thoughts.

4.5 Strategies to Counter Cognitive Avoidance

Section objectives:
- **Present strategies that are more effective than cognitive avoidance for dealing with fear of cancer recurrence:**
  – Cognitive restructuring (questioning the validity and usefulness of thoughts)
  – Planned worry time (planning a convenient moment for worrying instead of trying to drive away negative thoughts throughout the day)
  – Learning to tolerate unpleasant thoughts instead of trying to fight them off (quicksand and Aunt Irma metaphors)
  – Cognitive exposure (facing the worst possible future scenario)

4.5.1 Slide #9: Cognitive Restructuring

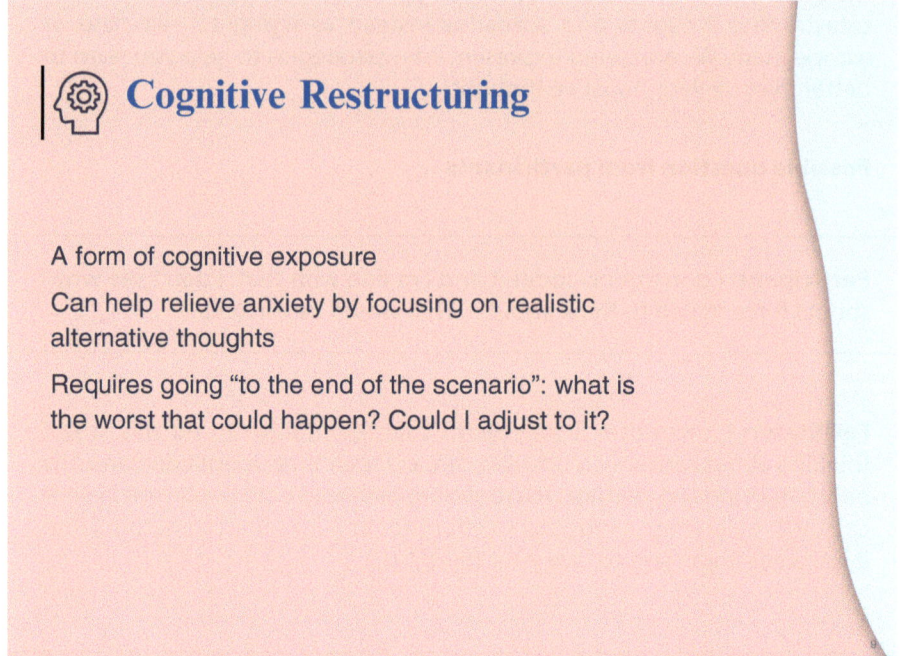

At this point, present some strategies that are generally more effective for dealing with negative thoughts. Start with cognitive restructuring, which was already explained during a previous session. You may ask participants if they remember some of the cognitive restructuring questions, such as: "What is the evidence that this thought is true? Is there another more likely explanation? What is the worst that could happen?" Explain that questioning the validity and usefulness of their thoughts and the resulting change in perspective may be enough to relieve their anxiety and reduce overwhelming emotions. After all, thinking about the worst-case scenario is a form of cognitive exposure. However, also tell them that if thoughts keep coming back or a catastrophic scenario remains in their mind despite their attempts at cognitive restructuring, they should try other strategies.

4.5.2 Slide #10: Planned "Worry Time"

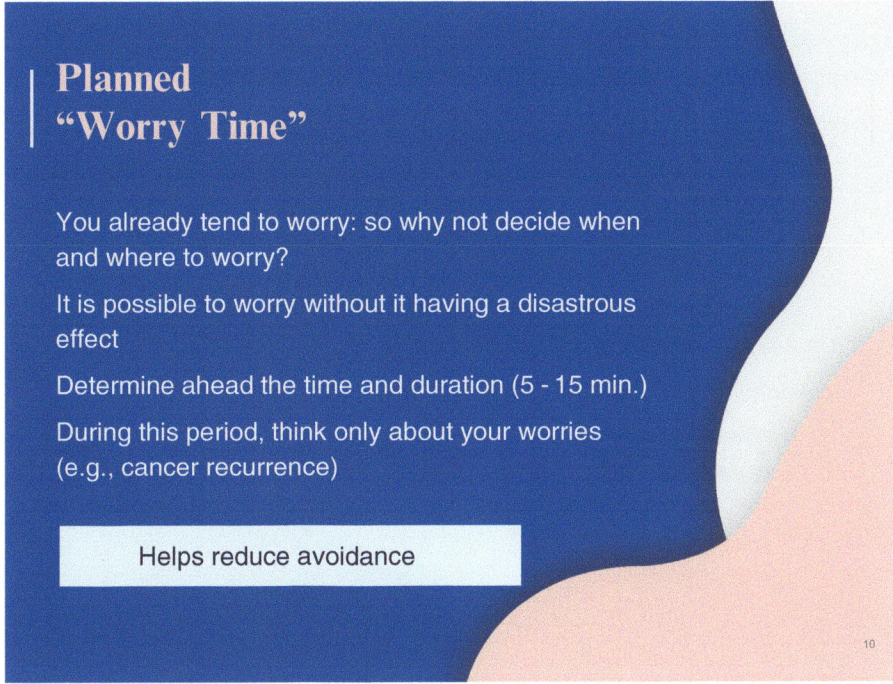

Facilitator: Anxious people tend to worry a lot throughout the day. Because their worries do not always arise at a good time (e.g. at work), they are forced to drive away these disturbing thoughts so they can continue to function. Alternatively, planned "worry time" is a time set in advance to deal with negative thoughts. Worry time involves a place and fixed period of 5–15 min that you must determine ahead. During this time, you will allow your worries to surface so you can face them. This means that each time that a concern comes to mind during the day, you tell yourself that it is not the right time and wait until your planned worry time to think about it. This is different from avoidance because the idea is to confront your thoughts, but later, at a predetermined time. This strategy allows you to face anxiety-inducing thoughts, therefore reducing avoidance. It also allows to gain some control over these types of thoughts by letting them surface at a convenient time for you. You already tend to worry, so why not decide when and where to worry? This strategy will help you see that you can worry without it having a disastrous effect. Moreover, planned worry time allows you to take a step back from your thoughts, which can help you see that they are just thoughts, not reality. In the end, you will probably worry a lot less.

4.5.3 Slide #11: Tolerating Negative Thoughts and Emotions

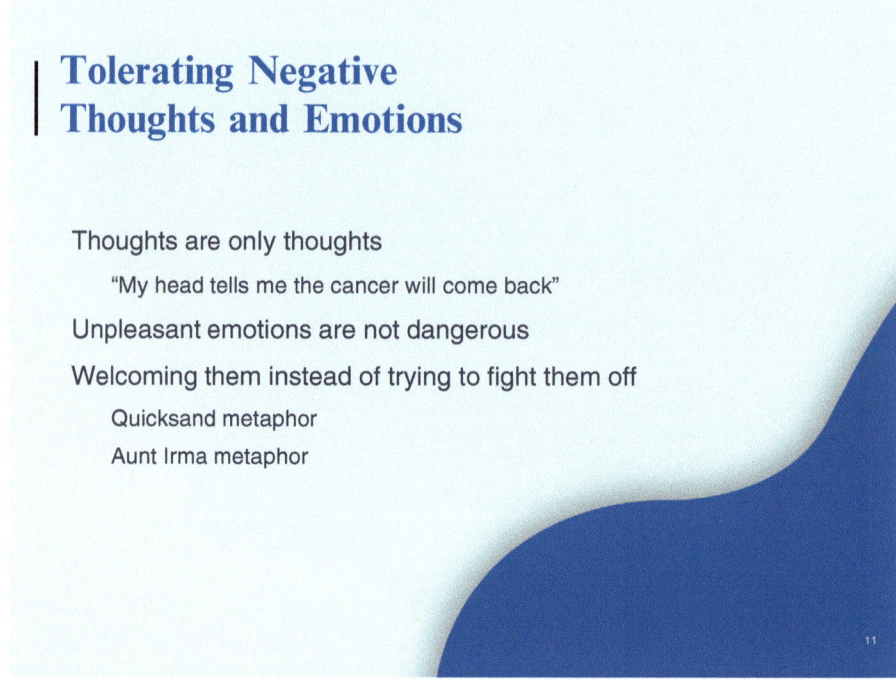

Next, highlight the importance of learning to tolerate negative thoughts and emotions. This involves realizing that thoughts are only thoughts, and the emotions generated by them are undoubtedly unpleasant but not dangerous. The idea here is not to make light of fear of cancer recurrence but rather to recognize that thoughts associated with it are just a product of the mind, not reality. More specifically, this involves welcoming unpleasant thoughts and emotions rather than trying to fight them off. In short, we have little control over our thoughts when they arise, but we can control our attitude towards them. Then, describe the quicksand metaphor.

4.5 Strategies to Counter Cognitive Avoidance

> **Facilitator:** When a person is stuck in quicksand, their natural reaction is to try to escape. By desperately raising one foot in an attempt to get themselves out of the sand, they only increase the pressure exerted by the other foot that is supporting the weight of their entire body, thus resulting in them sinking even deeper. Paradoxically, the only way to free themselves from the quicksand is to lie down because by increasing the contact area with the mud, the pressure produced by their body decreases, hence giving them a chance to float. In other words: They must stop fighting to get out. The same is true for negative emotions. An emotion is like a wave that comes and goes. You will never be overwhelmed permanently by a feeling: it is just a bad moment that will pass. So, it is best to welcome your emotions instead of trying to fight them.

You can also describe the Aunt Irma metaphor (Schoendorff, 2009) by telling them the following:

> **Facilitator:** Because cognitive avoidance is a rather abstract concept, we will illustrate it with the Aunt Irma metaphor. Perhaps you have an aunt who is kind of the black sheep of the family and a little unpleasant, and who you always hesitate to invite to family gatherings because she always puts a damper on the party by bringing up boring subjects or whining and complaining about everything. We are going to use the example of such an aunt, who we will call Irma. Imagine that you are planning a party at your place and invite your whole family, except Aunt Irma. You do not want her to be there. On the evening of the party, everyone is at your place having fun. Then, there is a knock at the door, and when you look out the window, you see Aunt Irma. You really wanted to avoid her showing up there, but there she is.

Next, ask participants what they would do in a similar situation. Listed below are various examples of answers they could give, along with suggested feedback for each one.

- **We could tell her that we can't welcome her because the house is already full**: Tell participants that this is indeed an option, that they could tell her that, unfortunately, she must leave. Another possibility would be to tell her that she is not welcome. Ask participants how they think Aunt Irma would react. Obviously, the risk with this option is that she becomes angry and starts to make a scene.

- **We could turn up the music and pretend that we don't hear her:** In this case, Aunt Irma is also likely to make a scene and perhaps even disturb the neighbours. Then, all the attention would be on Aunt Irma, and everyone would probably become uncomfortable. It is undoubtedly an option, but it would still ruin the party.
- **We let her in, but we monitor everything that she says to make sure that she is not being inappropriate**. Ask participants what impacts this attempt at control would have, including on themselves. Here, you may highlight that this option would also ruin their evening. Besides, they are unlikely to succeed in their attempt to control Aunt Irma's every move.
- **We let her in and enjoy our party**: Tell them that the good thing about this option is that their attention is not entirely focused on Aunt Irma. Of course, they would have preferred her to be somewhere else because they do not like her very much, but the impact on the party and themselves would be less significant than it would be with the other options.

> **Facilitator:** Basically, Aunt Irma represents the unpleasant thoughts and emotions that we sometimes have. Unfortunately, they will arise whether we like it or not. In a day, many unpleasant thoughts or feelings may surface, as much as you might like them to disappear. Given this fact, what is most important is your attitude towards such thoughts and emotions. You can try to fight them or pretend that they are not there, but despite your best efforts, you will inevitably end up paying a lot of attention to them, ultimately preventing you from enjoying life. Instead, you could try welcoming these thoughts or emotions (or Aunt Irma from our example) by tolerating their presence (even if it is difficult), while also focusing your attention on what is important to you (enjoying yourselves and your guests' company).

Next, ask participants if the explanations are clear so far and make sense to them. Tell them that the goal is not to make light of unpleasant thoughts and emotions, but instead to provide them with tools to better deal with them.

4.5.4 Slide #12: Cognitive Exposure

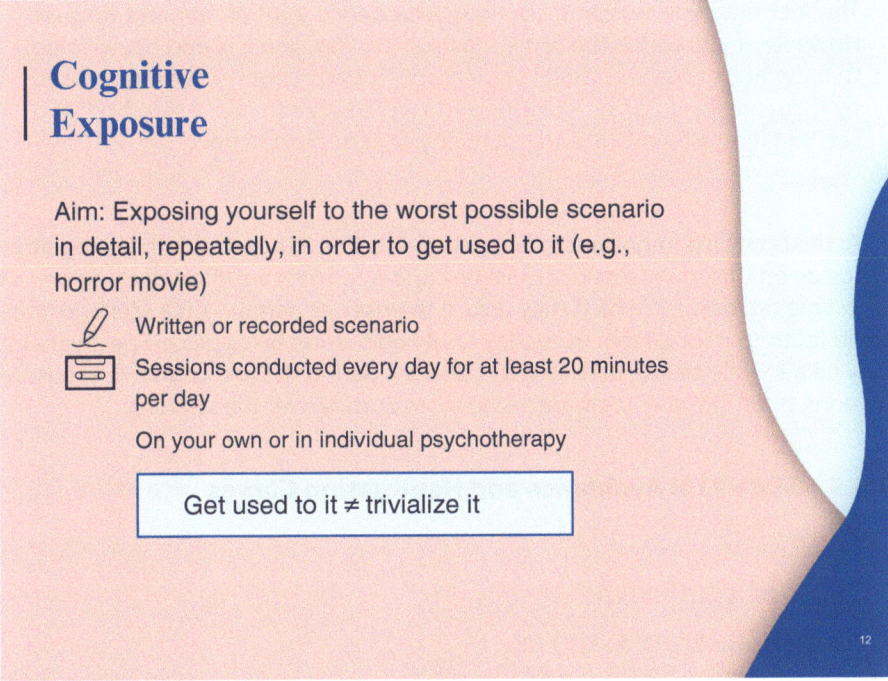

Finally, present the cognitive exposure strategy to participants. Tell them that it is usually conducted in individual (or group) psychotherapy to help people deal with any emotions that could arise. Still, they can also try this technique on their own. Specify that cognitive exposure involves facing the thought of the worst possible scenario that could occur (e.g. a cancer recurrence that ultimately leads to death, not having any support during such an ordeal, etc.). Some options could be to write down the worst possible scenario in detail, then read it again and again, or record themselves as they read it out loud and listen to the recording repeatedly.

Facilitator: It may seem counter-intuitive to force yourselves to think about what you fear the most, but just like with behavioural exposure, repeated exposure to catastrophic scenarios leads to habituation. As you face your thoughts, you will get used to them, and they will eventually stir up less unpleasant feelings. Again, by forcing yourselves to think about something upsetting, you will soon realize that thoughts are upsetting but not dangerous because nothing bad happens when you have them. Another beneficial effect of this strategy is that once a person has faced their worst-case scenario in their mind, they do not need to fight such thoughts anymore, which will provide some relief.

Facilitator: It is kind of like watching a horror movie over and over again. The first time you watch it, you may experience a lot of fear and disgust. However, if you watch the same movie every day, you will end up noticing that the horror scenes are still unpleasant to watch, but the feelings caused by them are less intense. Therefore, you will be able to take a step back and see that it is just a movie and not reality, that it is just fiction.

At this point, it is important to tell participants that if they decide to try cognitive exposure on their own, sessions must be conducted over a sufficiently long period each time (at least 20 min). If they record themselves narrating the scenario, they could listen to it for 20 min every day until habituation takes place. Specify that it may take a while before their anxiety subsides during the first cognitive exposure sessions, but it will eventually decrease more quickly over the sessions.

4.5.5 Slide #13: Avoidance and Habituation Curves

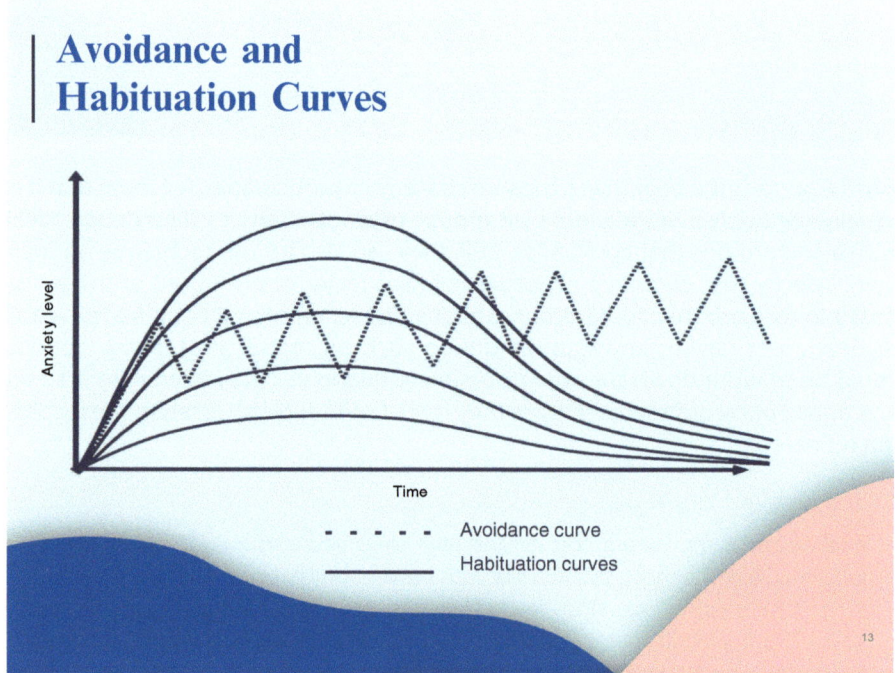

Referring to the habituation curve, mention that doing cognitive exposure only once a week, for example, is not enough and would be unnecessarily distressing. Also, specify that it is essential to include every possible detail in the scenario, as they would do for a movie scenario (e.g. the people present, the specific situation, the place, and the emotions felt).

Next, say the following to participants:

> **Facilitator:** Cognitive exposure does not mean trivializing the content of a scenario: it simply allows us to realize that it is just a scenario, not reality. Its content does not become less serious as we face it. But over time, the suspense disappears: "I know my horror story. In the end, I die." The goal is to get used to your thoughts about a specific scenario to reduce the intensity of the emotions you experience when you think about it.

Finally, tell participants that the goal was to propose various strategies that can help reduce cognitive avoidance. Mention that they could choose to use those that seem the most appropriate to their situation or work best for them.

4.6 Seeking Reassurance

Section objectives:

- **Explain what reassurance-seeking is to participants along with its consequences in the short and long term.**
- **Point out some clues that allow them to distinguish reassurance-seeking behaviours that are excessive from those that are adaptive.**
- **Remind participants that it is impossible to eliminate all doubt about a possible cancer recurrence and, as such, excessive reassurance-seeking is an ineffective strategy to deal with anxiety.**

4.6.1 Slides #14–15: The Vicious Circle of Fear of Recurrence and Reassurance Seeking: A Form of Avoidance

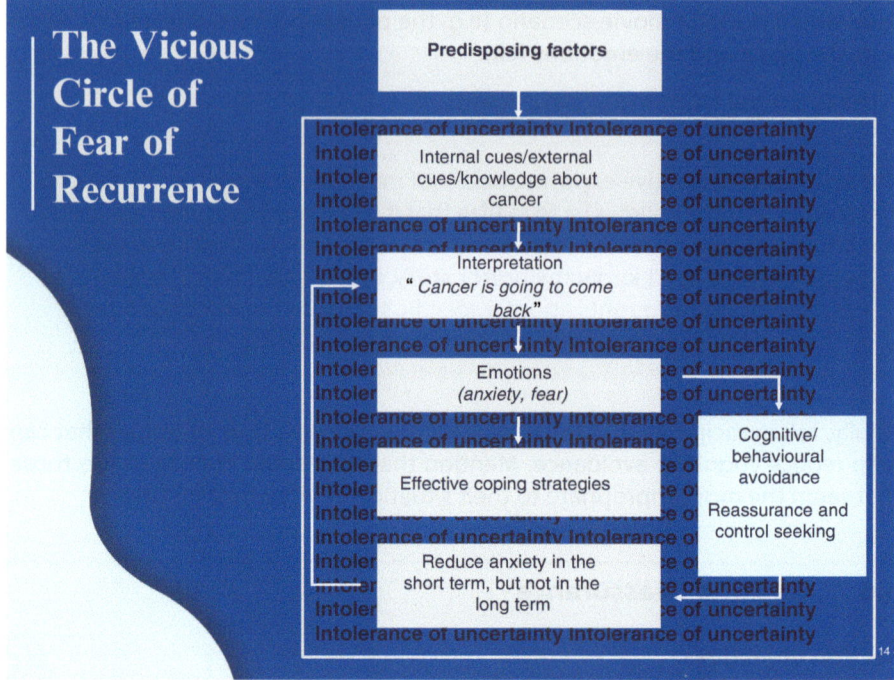

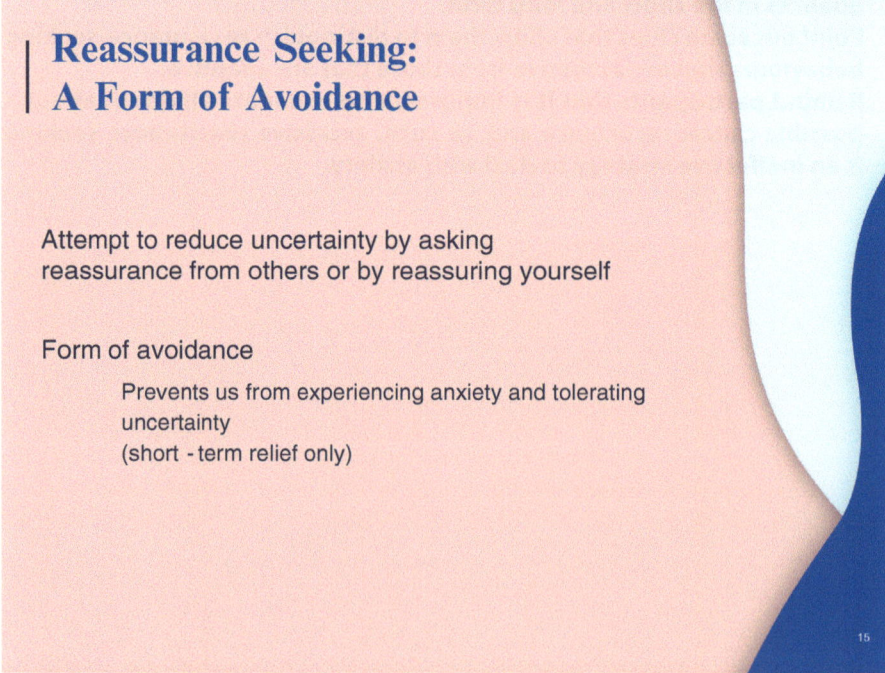

4.6 Seeking Reassurance

Facilitator: We will now discuss another element that appears in the same box as avoidance in our model: seeking reassurance and control. Seeking reassurance is a strategy often used by people to reduce their fear of cancer recurrence. It includes trying to reassure ourselves by thinking that everything will be fine and asking for reassurance from others, such as loved ones and health professionals. Obviously, it is appropriate to seek reassurance in some contexts, like when a new, intense, and persistent symptom appears. However, seeking excessive reassurance is a form of avoidance because it prevents us from experiencing anxiety and tolerating uncertainty. As with avoidance, reassurance may provide immediate relief, but this effect does not last very long. Have you noticed this, too?

4.6.2 Slide #16: Reassurance Behaviour Examples

Reassurance Behaviour Examples

- Repeated consultations with your doctor
- Asking for extra tests to be run
- Seeing several different health professionals
- Doing self-exams excessively
- Asking to be reassured by your loved ones
  "Promise me that everything is going to be fine"
- Trying to reassure yourself with ready-made thoughts
  "Everything will be fine"

Continue by giving participants a few examples of reassurance-seeking behaviours, such as repeated consultations with their doctor, seeing several different doctors for the same problem, asking for extra tests to be run, and so on. Tell them that many people would like to have tests done more often for this purpose exactly, that is, to be reassured. Likewise, to reduce their anxiety, many patients tend to ask the same questions to various health professionals, such as a nurse, a pharmacist, an oncologist, or even a psychologist. Again, the effect will only be short-lived. In addition, if what these various sources tell them is inconsistent, it will only cause even more anxiety. Patients can also do self-exams excessively: They check themselves to make sure they have no lumps that could be a sign of recurrence. Some patients may ask their loved ones to reassure themselves, to tell them that everything will be okay ("Promise me that everything is going to be fine"). Add that it is also common to try to reassure themselves with ready-made thoughts, such as: "Everything will be fine." Finally, ask participants if they recognize themselves in any of these reassurance-seeking behaviours that aim to eliminate uncertainty.

4.6.3 Slide #17: Reassurance: Yes, But to What Extent?

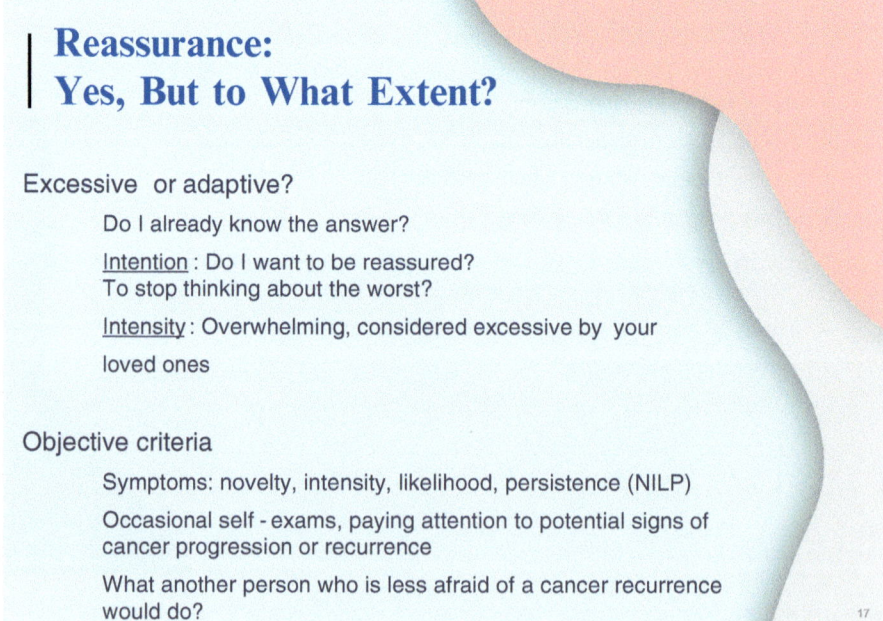

Conclude with the following:

> **Facilitator:** It is important to distinguish excessive reassurance-seeking behaviours from those that are adaptive. It is totally normal to ask your doctor questions; this behaviour is not always excessive. However, it may be excessive if you already know what your doctor will say because you have already asked them the same question, and you want them to repeat the answer because this will help relieve your anxiety. To determine whether a reassurance-seeking behaviour is adaptive or excessive, you must ask yourselves the following questions: What is my intention? Am I seeking new information or do I want to be reassured so I can stop thinking about the worst? How important are these reassurance requests in my life? As for symptoms, it can be helpful to use the objective criteria presented during the second session (NILP) to assess whether it would be relevant to seek medical attention. Of course, occasional self-exams and careful monitoring of potential signs of recurrence are good practices. The goal is not to become neglectful towards possible signs of recurrence but to find a certain balance. In this vein, it can be helpful to ask yourselves what another person with less fear of recurrence would do if they were in your shoes. For example, how many times a day, week, or month would they check themselves for signs of recurrence?

4.7 Seeking Control

Section objectives:

- **Present other types of behaviours that aim to increase the sense of control over the disease.**
- **Help participants understand the difference between changes in lifestyle habits that aim to improve quality of life versus those motivated by avoidance.**
- **Highlight that there is no such thing as an anti-cancer lifestyle, that scientific data are constantly evolving on factors influencing cancer, that it is important to have realistic goals with regards to lifestyle changes, and that pleasure is important in life.**

4.7.1 Slide #18: Seeking Control

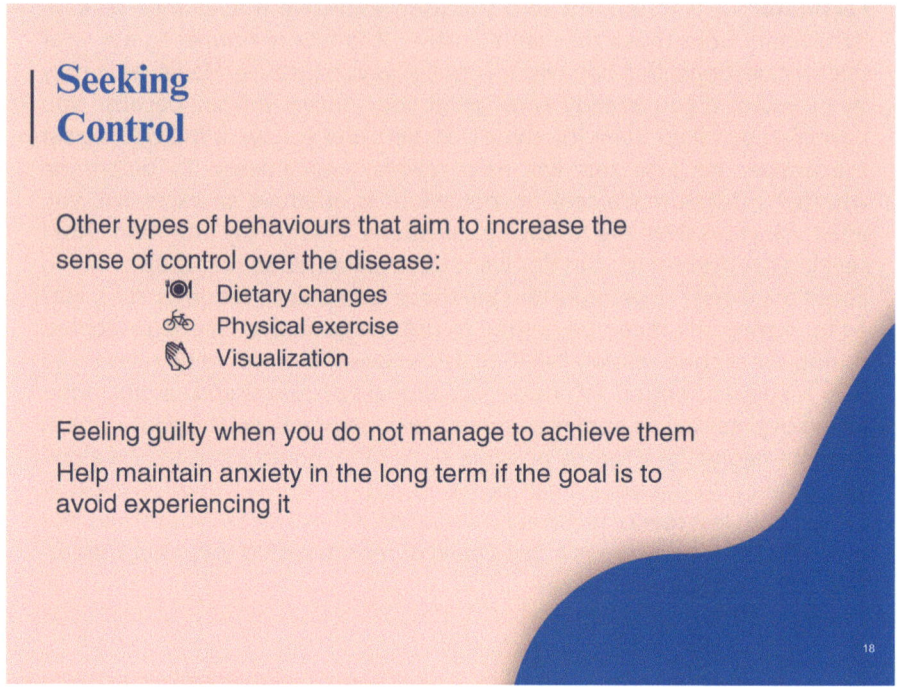

Continue by introducing the next topic, which is seeking control. This type of behaviour happens to be in the same box as avoidance and seeking reassurance in the fear of cancer recurrence model. Explain that patients often wonder what they could do to prevent cancer from coming back, especially during the post-treatment phase. As a result, many patients may drastically change some of their lifestyle habits, such as diet and exercise. They may even begin to practise activities that are promoted as beneficial to health, such as visualization (e.g. imagining their cells attacking and destroying cancer) to reduce the risk of the disease coming back.

Facilitator: Of course, starting to eat better, exercise, and practising meditation are not bad things as such. Health-wise, it can even be great to adopt such habits, and some of them may even help reduce the risk of cancer recurrence. Nevertheless, this type of change also often aims to reduce anxiety through seeking a sense of control over the disease. Hence, it can also be an avoidance strategy that helps maintain anxiety because we can never achieve a total sense of control; the things we do are never enough. For example, you may feel guilty about eating French fries, drinking a glass of wine, not exercising, or forgetting to practise visualization, regardless of all the efforts you made over the previous days. Drastic lifestyle changes may therefore be an attempt to control a risk over which you do not entirely have control. Do you recognize yourselves in any of these behaviour patterns? Remember what was discussed during the first session when we presented the multifactorial model of cancer, which consisted of a multitude of factors that can contribute to cancer. You may have some control over certain factors, but not over others.

4.7.2 Slide #19: Seeking Control

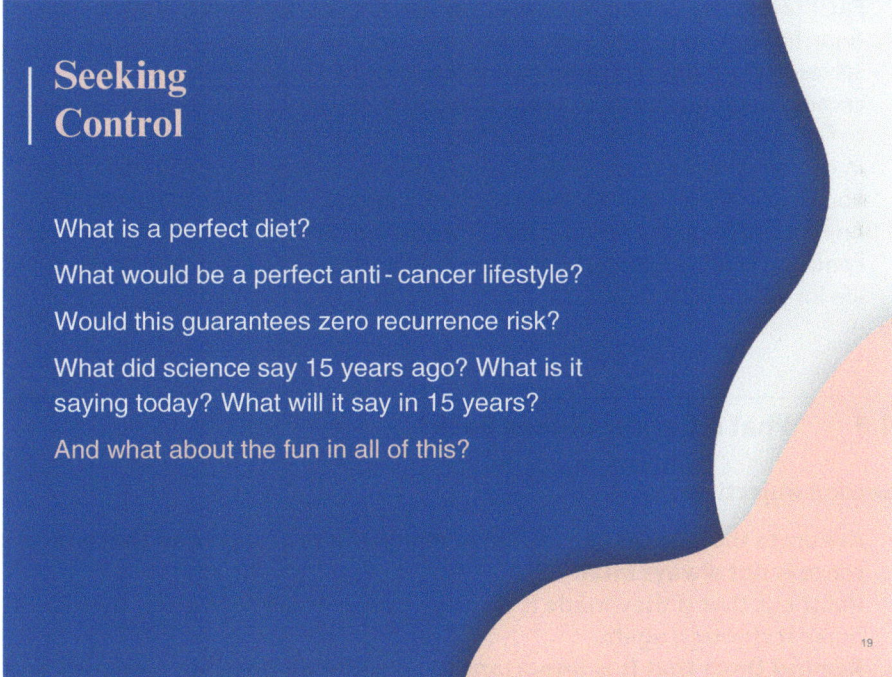

> **Facilitator:** What is also important to remember is that there is no magic food or food to be avoided at all costs that would completely eliminate the possibility of recurrence. The nutritional organization general recommendations are to eat a balanced diet with a lot of fruits, vegetables, and fibres, stop smoking, maintain a healthy body weight, and reduce a sedentary lifestyle by doing physical exercise. However, there are no specific standards to achieve. For example, there is no such thing as an anti-cancer diet.

Next, suggest that participants be realistic and flexible by doing what they feel like doing without turning it into strict rules to follow as this could lead them to feel guilty when they do not stick to them. Also, specify that there is no such thing as an anti-cancer lifestyle that guarantees zero recurrence risk. To support your point, point out that many people who developed cancer already had excellent lifestyle habits. Finally, emphasize that constant progress in science always leads to discovering a miracle food that is later found to either have no actual effect or even be harmful to other health conditions. In short, the goal is to find a lifestyle that is suited to their values and help improve their well-being and quality of life without becoming rigid about it.

> **Facilitator:** My last point focuses on fun. If it is important to you to continue to drink wine with your meal, then continue to do so. Depriving yourselves of the things you enjoy will not necessarily prevent the disease from coming back. Make any changes that you both want and feel able to make to feel your best and have the best possible quality of life. There is no point in deciding never to eat junk food or drink alcohol again if you know that you would not be able to make such changes. It would just make you feel unnecessarily guilty, and besides, it would not ensure that cancer will not come back. An oncologist once told one of our patients, "I didn't save your life for you to stop living!"

4.8 What If Cancer Comes Back?

Section objectives:

- **Reiterate that cancer can evolve in many different ways and that a recurrence is not always fatal.**
- **Point out that if they made it through cancer treatment once, they could make it through again.**
- **Remind them that it is important to consider all possible scenarios and maintain realistic hope.**

4.8.1 Slide #20: What If Cancer Comes Back?

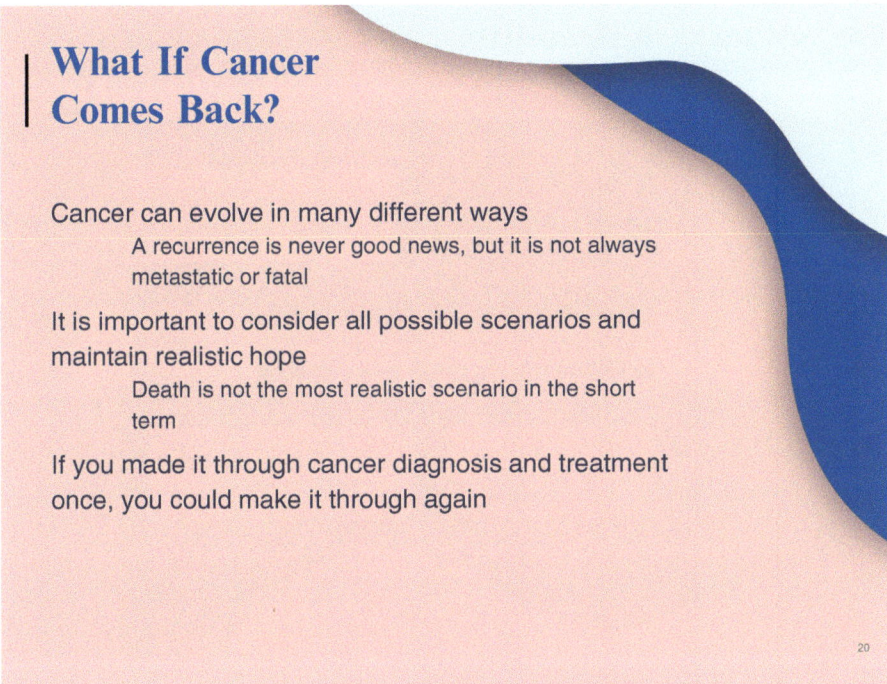

Begin the next section on the possibility of a recurrence as follows:

Facilitator: We will now focus on the question that we usually wish to avoid as much as possible after being treated for cancer: "What if it comes back?" Our goal here is to help you interpret more flexibly what such a scenario would involve. Often, people with a high fear of recurrence tend to associate cancer recurrence with death. Fortunately, this is not always the case in reality. Remember that cancer can evolve in many different ways, and this is true for all types of cancer. Of course, being told that cancer has come back is never good news to receive, but a recurrence is not always metastatic or fatal. Indeed, it is important to remember that, just as for an initial cancer diagnosis, a recurrence can also be effectively treated and controlled and lead to remission. Also, remember that realistic optimism involves considering all possible scenarios while hoping for the best possible outcome. By remembering that cancer can evolve in many different ways and challenging the idea that recurrence means death, it becomes easier to have hope that death is not the most realistic scenario in the short term, which makes recurrence seem less catastrophic.

4.8.2 Slide #21: Recurrence ≠ Death

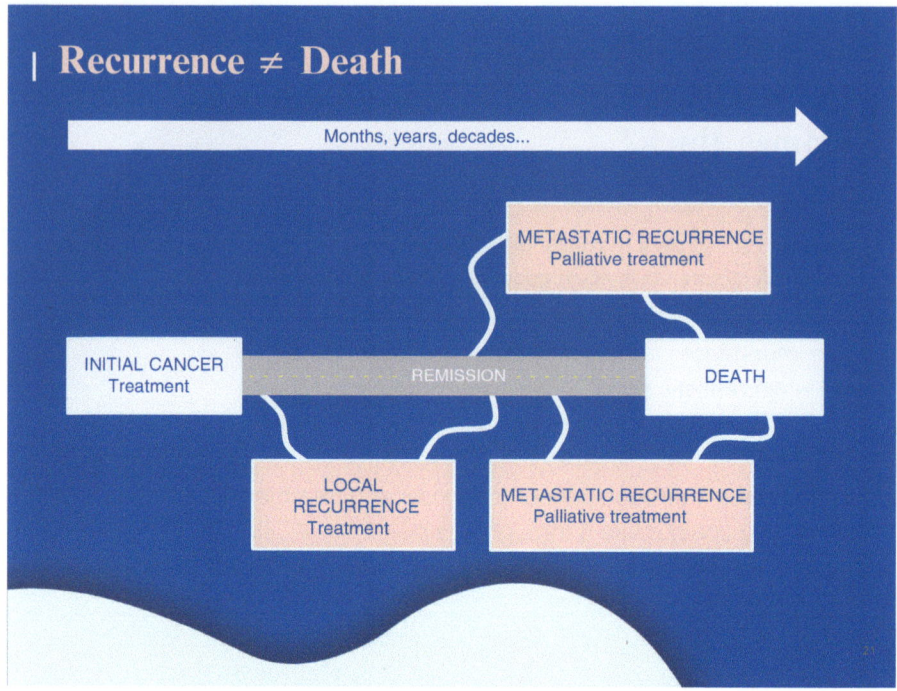

At this point, you can again show the figure illustrating the different possible courses of the disease again. You can also give one or a few examples of patients you know who were treated for a recurrence many years ago and are still alive today.

Continue by returning to the previous slide and highlighting that patients are often afraid of recurrence because it can be fatal, but also because they do not want to have to go through everything they went through after their initial diagnosis. Tell them that you understand very well that the idea of cancer coming back and undergoing treatment again is not very encouraging. Sometimes, some patients can even be convinced that they will not have the strength to get through it a second time.
Continue by asking them the following questions:

> **Facilitator:** What resources helped you get through your cancer experience? Tell me about your personal resources and the help you received from the people around you.

> **Participant:** My sister helped me a lot. She prepared meals for me, took care of my children when I was not feeling well, and listened when I was having a rough time.

Participant: My strength of character is what helped get me through it.

Facilitator: Interesting! Now, I would like you to consider the following question: which resources were there for you when you were first diagnosed and treated for cancer and would still be there for you if cancer came back?

Participant: My sister would certainly still be there for me.

Participant: In my case, everything I read and already know about cancer would help me.

Facilitator: Could we conclude that you would have the necessary resources to get through the cancer experience for a second time, even if we can agree that it would be best if cancer did not come back?

Participant: Yes, probably, especially now that we know what help is available to us.

Participant: I'm afraid of putting my loved ones through such an ordeal again.

Facilitator: Yes, I understand. However, aren't there also resources that could help them face cancer with you, and wouldn't they still have access to them if cancer were to come back?

Point out to participants that if they managed to make it through a cancer diagnosis and treatment once, they will probably be able to make it through again, though such an experience would obviously not be desirable or enjoyable. Also, tell them that when thinking about cancer recurrence, it is common to imagine all the subsequent steps that would have to be taken, making it seem like a mountain to climb all at once (treatment, side effects, impact on their lives, etc.). In reality, they would go through those steps one at a time as they did for their initial diagnosis and treatment. It is also essential for them to realize that they would probably not undergo the same treatment and experience the same side effects as the first time (perhaps even less of them?), or know how to manage them better (e.g. fatigue). Next, tell them that, fortunately, the initial feeling of dread about undergoing new treatment tends to fade over time. In short, help them see that humans are very resilient in the face of adversity. Finally, ask them what they think about the ideas that were presented and whether they believe that considering recurrence from such a perspective is helpful.

4.9 Redefining Life Goals

Section objectives:

- **Help participants understand that it is crucial to have life goals (they give purpose in life).**
- **Explain that it is always possible to have life goals that are adapted to their values and capacities.**
- **Highlight that the important thing is not necessarily to achieve life goals but to take action to bring them closer to what is important to them.**
- **Propose exercises to help them reflect on life goals that are meaningful to them and enrich their lives.**

4.9.1 Slide #22: The Importance of Life Goals

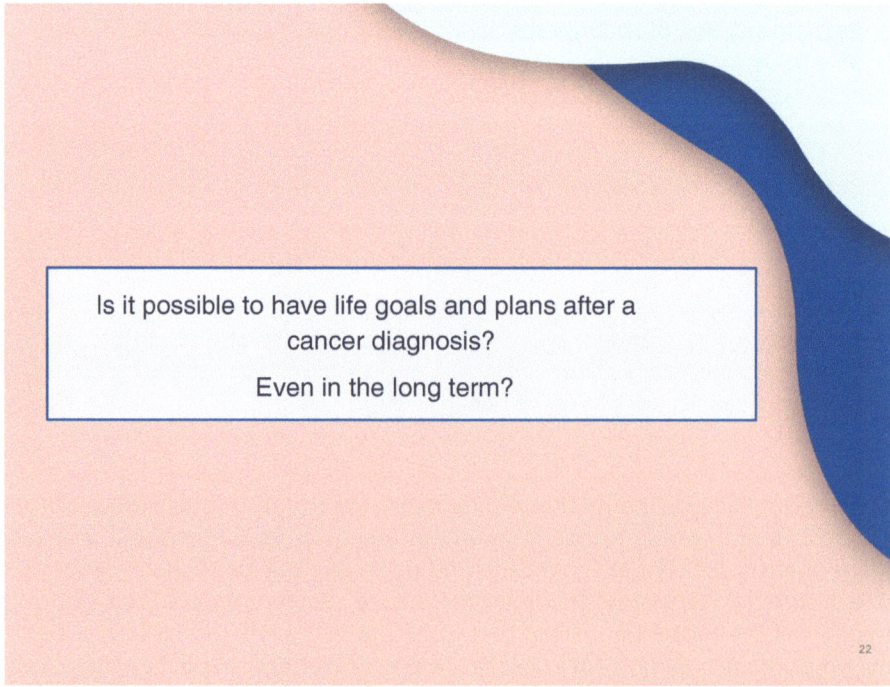

4.9 Redefining Life Goals

Here is a possible discussion with participants on this topic:

Facilitator: Is it possible to have life goals and plans after a cancer diagnosis? Even in the long term? Does anyone here find that the possibility of the disease coming back keeps them from planning for the future or that it affects their thoughts about it?

Participant: I would say that in the beginning, I could not make plans beyond the next two months. Now, my mental calendar is open for the next year. However, I opened it gradually: I went from two to three months, then from three to four, and so forth.

Participant: I now agree to things that are scheduled in the next few months. I'm nervous about saying yes, but I already found a solution by telling myself that if worse comes to worst, someone else will be able to do what I was supposed to do, and this helps calm me.

Facilitator: Exactly! You have all shared some very interesting points! In the end, and this is the case for everyone, cancer or no cancer: if something prevents us from achieving a goal, it's always possible for us to readjust it. This is just as true now as it was before you had cancer. For example, anyone planning a trip can never be sure that it will take place because various obstacles may stand in the way, such as illness, injury, lack of money, and so on.

Participant: It's just that before, we didn't think about it.

Facilitator: Exactly! The same thing was true before, but this didn't keep you from making plans for the future, right?

Here is another possible type of discussion that you could have with participants:

Facilitator: What are the benefits of having life goals?

Participant: It's nice to have some.

Facilitator: Why?

Participant: Living life without a purpose or goal is kind of boring. It's just robotic.

Facilitator: Indeed, we need reasons to get up in the morning. So, does it really matter whether the goals we set for ourselves are achieved or not? If we take the example of beginning a long study program, what would make such a goal beneficial? Is it only when we get a diploma at the end of the program that we are happy and satisfied with ourselves, or is it also possible to feel satisfaction daily while following the program?

Participant: I think so. I would probably experience it like that. Having different courses and professors would be enriching on a daily basis. For example, I don't even work in my field of study, but my studies allowed me to meet my friends and have fun.

Facilitator: Indeed, the pleasure we draw from projects can also be experienced along the road we take to make them happen. Sometimes, you may set limits for yourselves for health reasons and avoid making long-term goals because you don't know what the future has in store for you. At the same time, you should remember that just because you're not sure whether you will complete the project or not does not mean that you should stop setting goals for yourself. The process in itself is enjoyable, not only its result. And a life without goals is likely to lead to depressive symptoms in the long term.

4.9.2 Slides #23–24: The Case of Alfred

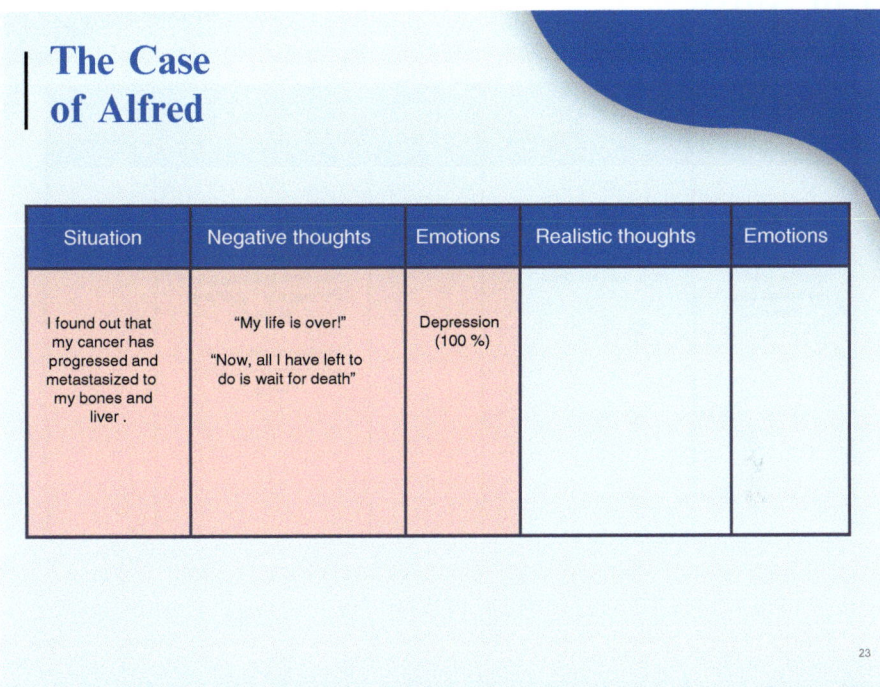

Continue by illustrating the case of Alfred, a patient who recently found out that his cancer has progressed and metastasized to his bones and liver. Obviously, this situation stirs up many negative thoughts, such as: "My life is over," "Now, all I have left to do is wait for death," as well as painful emotions (depression 100%).

The Case of Alfred

Situation	Negative thoughts	Emotions	Realistic thoughts	Emotions
I found out that my cancer has progressed and metastasized to my bones and liver.	"My life is over!" "Now, all I have left to do is wait for death"	Depression (100 %)	"Indeed, my life expectancy is limited, but I'm still alive. I still have time to carry out plans that are important to me." "Waiting to die would only depress me even more."	Depression (30 %)

Facilitator: We are going to do an exercise to help Alfred find realistic thoughts that could help him experience his situation differently. Does anyone here have any ideas of alternative thoughts or other ways of seeing things after receiving such bad news?

Participant: I would say that it's important to make the most of the life I have left, to live it to the fullest. We never know when everything will come to an end. In our case, it could be tomorrow, or it could be in 10 or 20 years. So, we have to make the most of it every day. That's what we should tell ourselves.

4.9 Redefining Life Goals

Facilitator: So, you're saying that it's important to continue to have dreams and make the most of life regardless of what lies ahead. Excellent! Alfred could tell himself: "Indeed, my life expectancy is limited, but I'm still alive. I still have time to carry out plans that are important to me. Also, waiting to die would only depress me even more." So, with realistic thinking, Alfred is obviously not happier about his prognosis, but this attitude helps give him a little more perspective by bringing him to focus on what is truly important to him. This leads me to ask you another question. In Alfred's situation, is it still possible to have life goals? If so, to what extent?

Participant: I know someone who had pancreatic cancer. He has since died, but when he found out about it, he was told that he probably had about two months left to live. However, his daughter was planning on getting married six months later. He really wanted to be there for her wedding, so it became a goal for him. In the end, he managed to make it to her wedding!

Facilitator: So, he allowed himself to hope that he could be there, even if he was not sure that it would be possible. This is a perfect example of realistic optimism. And maintaining hope that he could make it to his daughter's wedding probably helped him feel better in his last months.

Continue by saying the following to participants:

Facilitator: In short, the important thing with life goals is not necessarily to achieve them, but to reflect on them and take action to move closer towards them because they help make life more enjoyable and satisfying. It's also possible to change your life goals so that they better fit your reality. For example, a person diagnosed with an advanced form of cancer will probably have to change their initial life goals. Consider the example of a person who planned to backpack through Europe, which becomes unrealistic due to the pain and fatigue related to cancer. They could change their goal to make it more realistic and possible to enjoy by going on a short, organized trip, for example.

If you wish, you can tell the story of the following case:

> **Facilitator:** Now, I will tell you about a man who went through a situation similar to Alfred's and decided to seek psychological counselling. As the session began, he talked about how several years ago, he was given only six months to live. He said that he hoped that the psychologist could help him learn to live again. This man had completely stopped doing all the activities that he enjoyed and had just started waiting to die, which still had not happened after all those years. He had stopped working and quit his bowling league. He practically never saw his friends and was depressed. Obviously, it is exceptional for a person to outlive their prognosis to such an extent, but it is still something that we see now and then. Indeed, we see more and more people who live many years with metastatic cancer. So, if we stop living when we are told that our cancer cannot be cured, a lot of time can go by. This is why it is so important to have life goals even when our life expectancy is reduced. In short, it is always good to have life goals and to be able to adjust them to our reality, if necessary. The worst that could happen is that we do not manage to achieve our goals, but isn't that much less harmful than keeping ourselves from making the most of our lives every day?

4.9.3 Slide #25: Redefining Life Goals (Step 1)

Redefining Life Goals (Step 1)

Unconstrained goals "magic wand"	Current objectives
Backpacking trip through Europe	Organized trip to Europe
Buy a cabin by a lake	Rent a cabin, next summer
Learn to play the piano	Learning new things
Make a photo album	Make a photo album
Running a marathon	Be physically active
Getting closer to my grandchildren	Getting closer to my grandchildren

Next, suggest an exercise for the participants to do. First (first column), they may consider the following questions: "What have I always wanted to do that I have not done yet? What are my dreams? If I had a magic wand that could eliminate cancer, what would I want to do?" Continue by proposing that they identify among their goals those that are still achievable. They could write these goals down in the "Current goals" column. In this column, they could also write down an adapted version of their unachievable goals (like the backpacking trip to Europe mentioned previously). Another example is that a person may not have the financial means to buy a cabin by a lake as they have always dreamed of doing, but they could still rent one for a few weeks during the summer.

4.9.4 Slide #26: Redefining Life Goals (Step 2)

Redefining Life Goals (Step 2)

My new life goals	Short-term goals	Medium-term goals	Long-term goals
Getting closer to my grandchildren	Invite my grandchildren over for dinner more often	Spending the next summer holiday with them	Moving to the same city as them

Next, tell the participants that a key aspect of this exercise is to break each life goal down into several goals for the short, medium, and long terms. This will help them take action, and breaking down each goal into several smaller ones will make the experience more quickly satisfying. Specify that the time frame is relative for each person, which means that six months can represent a short-term goal for one person and a long-term goal for another, depending on their own perspective and life expectancy. Finally, mention that there is no predetermined end for which they must plan: their goals can extend beyond their prognosis as long as they remain realistic.

Take the time to look at the example of wanting to get closer to one's grandchildren by breaking it down into concrete goals. Tell the participants that a person with this goal may start by setting a short-term goal (e.g. inviting their grandchildren over for dinner more often), then a medium-term goal (e.g. spending their next summer holiday with them), and finally, a long-term goal (e.g. moving to the same city as them).

4.9.5 Slide #27: Avenues for Reflection

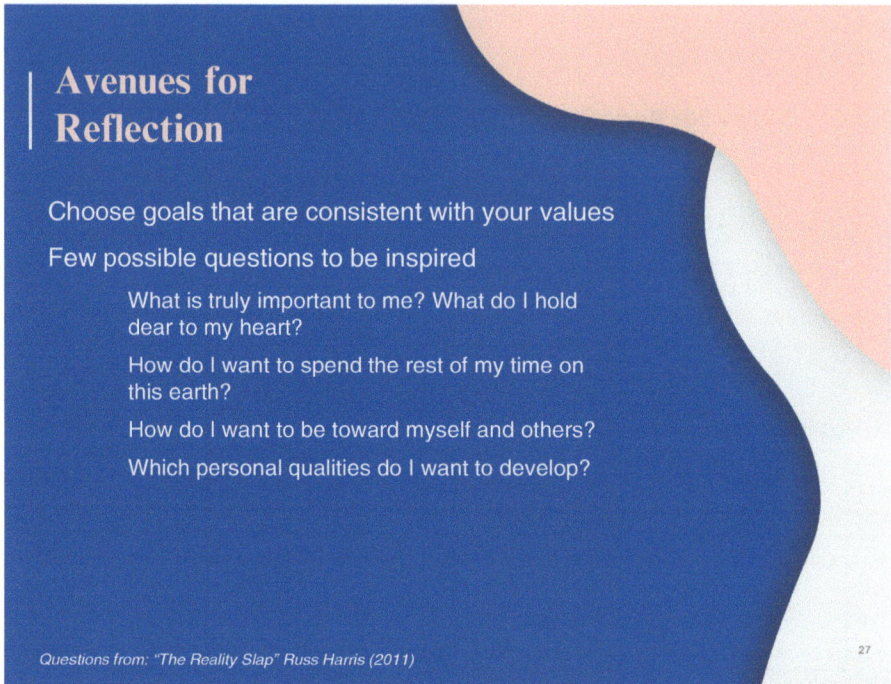

At this point, present a list of questions that can also be found on the exercise sheet. Explain that these questions are meant to inspire them throughout their thought process. While this may be very natural for some people, it may be more difficult for others to identify their values and what is important to them because they are not used to asking themselves these kinds of questions.

Facilitator: These questions are meant to help you choose goals that are consistent with your values and that will give your life meaning. Here are a few possible questions: "What is truly important to me? What do I hold dear to my heart? How do I want to spend the rest of my time on this earth? How do I want to be towards myself and others? What qualities do I want to develop?" As you can see, projects do not necessarily have to "cost" something: They can also be actions that you want to take so you can make the most of life and grow as a person.

4.10 Slide #28: End of Session Discussion

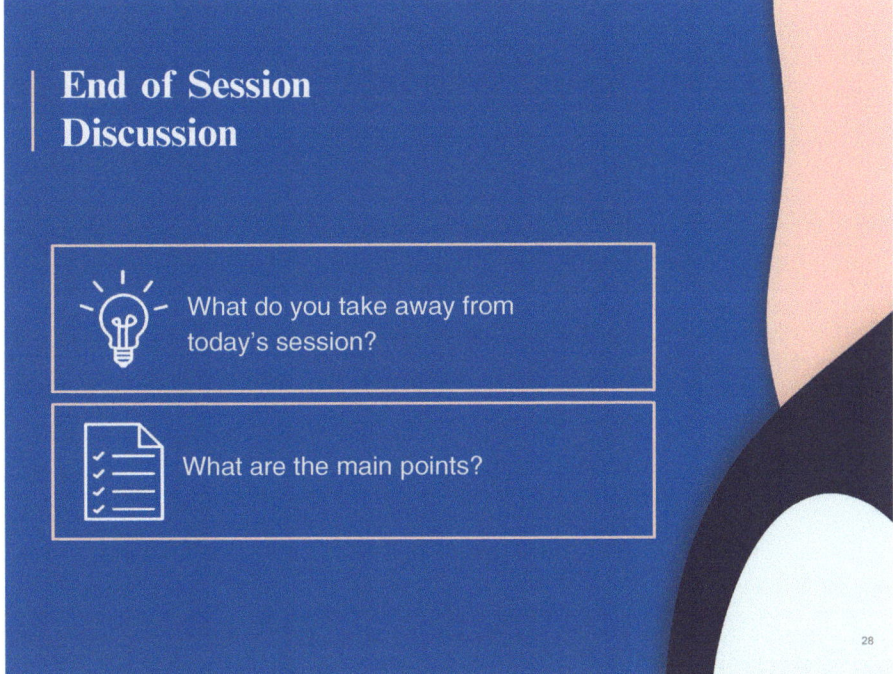

Ask the participants what they took away from the session (two to four main points). Ask them about their impressions, appreciation, and comments and whether they have any questions about the material presented today.

4.11 Slide #29: Tools in Brief

Tools in Brief

Issues	Solutions
Tendency to drive away negative thoughts (cognitive avoidance)	Cognitive restructuring (grid) Planned worry time Welcoming thoughts and "letting them pass" instead of trying to fight them off Cognitive exposure to the worst-case scenario
Seeking reassurance	Avoid asking for reassurance and learn to tolerate uncertainty Use objective criteria (NILP) to evaluate symptoms Ask myself what a person who is less afraid of recurrence would do
Seeking control	Seeking balance, well-being, and pleasure instead of control at all costs (e.g., food)
Trouble planning for the future	Redefining life goals

Summarize the main strategies discussed during the session to deal effectively with certain issues they may face.

4.12 General Review of the Psychotherapy Group

4.12.1 Slide #30: Conclusion

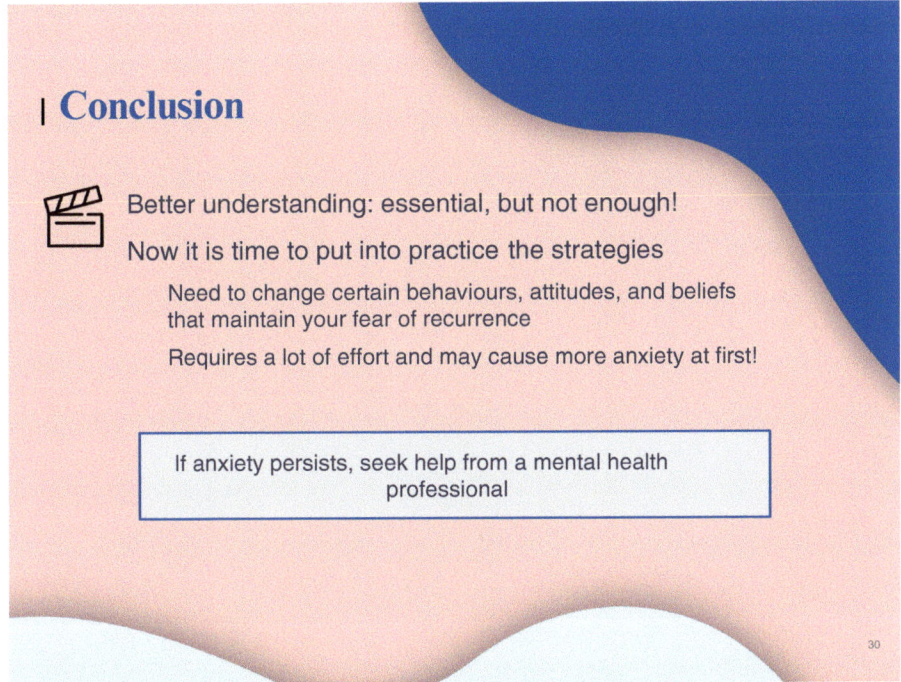

Ask participants what they took away from the four group sessions. Also, ask them about how they appreciated the program: What did they like more? Less? What helped them? Do they have any suggestions that could help improve the program?

Next, mention that it is important to understand why they are anxious about cancer recurrence and to know which strategies may maintain this fear and which ones they should use instead, but it is not enough. Explain that the next step (if it has not been done already) is to try to change certain harmful behaviours or attitudes identified during the sessions with the proposed tools. Emphasize that this will demand effort, especially when using the exposure strategy that generates anxiety at first but offers benefits in the long term. Ask participants to identify the next step in their journey to reduce their fear of cancer recurrence.

It is essential to mention that if their anxiety persists or remains a problem, and they find it difficult to apply the various suggested strategies, they might want to consider receiving individual psychotherapy.

Before concluding, make sure that the participants do not have any other questions or comments. Finally, thank them for their involvement and participation in the psychotherapy group.

Reference

Schoendorff, B. (2009). *Faire face à la souffrance, choisir la vie plutôt que la lutte avec la Thérapie d'Acceptation et d'Engagement*. Retz.

Part II

Psychotherapy Group on Fear of Cancer Recurrence: Participant's Manual

Session No. 1

5

5.1 What Is Fear of Recurrence?

5.1.1 Fear of Recurrence: Is It Normal or Not?

Fear of cancer recurrence is believed to affect, to varying degrees and at different times, almost everyone who has had cancer. This can be explained in part by the impossibility to predict who will or will not be cured of this disease marked by uncertainty. The ability to cope with the unpredictable nature of cancer varies greatly from one person to another. Some people even have what is called an "intolerance of uncertainty," which makes it extremely difficult for them to deal with the probabilities, such as those communicated to them by their oncologists: "Your chances of not having a recurrence are 85%." Since the probability of being cured is never 100%, these people are more likely to experience anxiety about a possible cancer recurrence.

Fear of recurrence is one of the most frequently reported issues by people having been treated for cancer. According to the definition adopted by a group of international experts, fear of cancer recurrence is defined as "fear, worry, or concern that cancer may come back or progress" (Lebel et al., 2016). This fear may emerge during the care trajectory and the period following the end of treatment, and last for many years. Levels of fear of recurrence vary greatly from one person to another. Many patients report worrying little about recurrence, except in the days or weeks before their medical exams and follow-ups. At these times, fear of recurrence tends to become more intense. Usually, it subsides after receiving test results that indicate an absence of signs of progression or recurrence of the disease. However, for a small number of people, the fear that cancer will come back can be very intense, even when their results indicate an absence of signs of progression. This fear can last for months or even years and it significantly affects their daily functioning. They will constantly have the disease on their mind despite their best efforts to stop thinking about it. In such cases, fear of recurrence is considered problematic because it causes intense distress, is overwhelming and/or persistent, and interferes with the person's functioning in different areas of their life.

Certain factors increase the risk of having a high level of fear of cancer recurrence, such as experiencing several side effects or physical symptoms following treatment, some aspects related to personality (e.g. having a lower tolerance to uncertainty), sociodemographic characteristics (being younger, being a woman), and having previously suffered from an anxiety disorder. While these factors may make some people more likely to develop a fear of recurrence, they alone are not enough to trigger and maintain it. Surprisingly, the intensity of the fear is not necessarily proportional to the real risk of recurrence. A person who has an excellent prognosis may still be strongly tormented by the idea that cancer could come back, whereas another person with a poorer prognosis may experience little fear.

5.1.2 Understanding the Vicious Circle of Fear of Recurrence

> *Julian is a 37-year-old man with testicular cancer. He describes himself as an anxious person with a tendency to worry excessively since he was a teenager. Since his diagnosis, he has been extremely vigilant to any new physical sensations (e.g. stomach pain) and reacts strongly when he hears an advertisement or a report on cancer in the media. His medical follow-up appointments are no picnic, partly because they are reminders that cancer could come back. Of course, this stirs up many emotions in him, including a great deal of anxiety. He also feels irritable, does not sleep well, and often feels like his stomach is in knots. To calm his anxiety, Julian developed a few strategies. He examines himself every time he goes to the bathroom to make sure that cancer has not "attacked" the other testicle. He also calls his nurse navigator regularly to check whether a symptom is normal or not. Finally, he tries to avoid everything that reminds him of the disease as much as possible. For example, when a friend asks him about his cancer, he automatically changes the subject.*

Do you think Julian is using the right strategies to deal with his fear of recurrence? If so, how can we explain the fact that his fear persists? To help you better understand this phenomenon, we elaborated an explanatory model of fear of cancer recurrence.

5.1 What Is Fear of Recurrence?

Explanatory model of fear of cancer recurrence

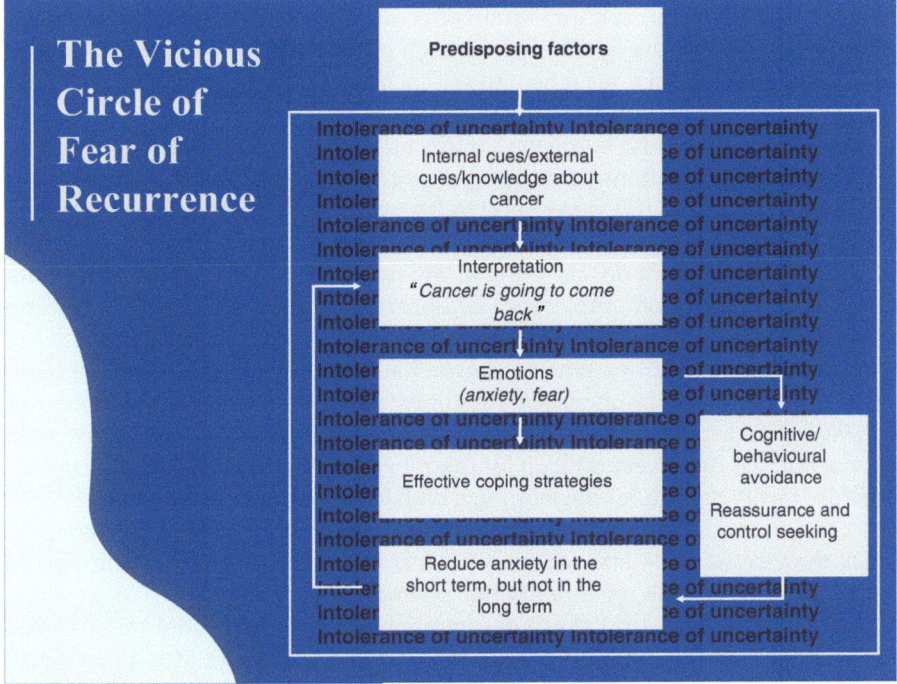

Fear of cancer recurrence is maintained over time through the development of a vicious circle. This vicious circle is activated by either internal cues (physical sensations such as pain) or external cues (medical appointments, information in the media, conversations with family and friends), and is influenced by your knowledge about cancer in general and about your specific type of cancer. Indeed, when we do not know whether a symptom is a sign of recurrence, we are more likely to worry about it. Symptoms that are especially likely to trigger fear of recurrence are those experienced before receiving the initial cancer diagnosis, but not exclusively. These internal and external cues then give rise to different thoughts, interpretations, and negative or even catastrophic perceptions (e.g. "Cancer is going to come back"), which, in turn, generate unpleasant emotions such as anxiety, fear, guilt, helplessness, sadness, or anger. In Julian's case, the vicious circle started with a stomach ache (internal cue) that he interpreted as a clear sign of cancer recurrence, which then caused him to become very anxious.

When faced with such a high level of anxiety, people will use all kinds of strategies to try to reduce it, some of which may be effective and others less so. Julian decided to call his nurse navigator to ask her if his stomach ache was normal. When she told him that it was not a worrisome symptom, Julian felt reassured, which led him to believe that his anxiety management strategy (calling his nurse navigator) was effective. However, this is not quite true. The use of strategies such as seeking reassurance (like in Julian's case), behavioural avoidance (e.g. avoiding reading or talking about cancer), or cognitive avoidance (e.g. avoiding thinking about cancer) can indeed be effective, but only in the short term. We will explain why in more detail in a later section. For now, remember that Julian's checking behaviours (i.e. his repeated self-examinations), his constant search for reassurance from healthcare professionals, and his efforts to avoid thinking about cancer are harmful in the long term and will instead maintain his fear over time. Indeed, the next time Julian has a physical symptom, he will again become very anxious and feel the same need to be reassured, which will again activate the vicious circle of fear of recurrence.

If you look at the model closely, you will notice an important concept in the background. It is called "intolerance of uncertainty." Anxious people, including those who have high levels of fear of cancer recurrence, tend to be intolerant of (or allergic to) uncertainty. When a person has this characteristic, they are quite likely to feel anxiety in uncertain situations such as cancer. For example, not knowing for sure what the future holds for them medically (*"Will cancer come back or not?"*) is often very difficult for them to bear. This individual characteristic provides fertile ground for developing a high level of fear of recurrence.

In this program, you will get to learn new and more effective strategies to block the vicious circle and reduce your fear of cancer recurrence, and also to help you cope with the uncertainty that characterizes cancer.

First, we shall focus on the "Interpretation" box of the model (refer to the explanatory model described previously). Although we have little power over the internal and external cues that may trigger the vicious circle, it is possible to learn to interpret them differently and therefore limit any negative emotions that may arise in response to certain interpretations of these cues. First, we will discuss the widely held belief that thoughts have the power to influence the course of cancer.

5.2 Can Thoughts Influence Cancer?

5.2.1 Beliefs About the Influence of Psychological Factors on Cancer

It is human nature to wish to understand what happens to us, why cancer appeared. However, it is rarely possible to know the exact causes of a disease such as cancer, which can be troubling. Cancer is a complex disease, and in most cases, its causes remain unknown to this day. Like many other chronic conditions, cancer is a multifactorial disease. In other words, there is no single etiology (cause) of cancer. Indeed, it is a combination of risk factors that, together, increase the possibility of developing cancer. These factors also vary from one person to another. For example, breast cancer may have mainly a genetic origin in some women, and in others, it may be linked more to hormonal factors and lifestyle habits.

Therefore, there is no single "recipe" for developing cancer, just as there is no single recipe for cake. Many ingredients are required, and their nature can vary from one person to another. Moreover, cancer is not just one disease: there are over 200 types of cancer, each with their own characteristics and determinants. Finally, remember that we still have a lot to learn about the causes of cancer. The following model illustrates this variety of factors, of which many have yet to be demonstrated:

Multifactorial model of cancer

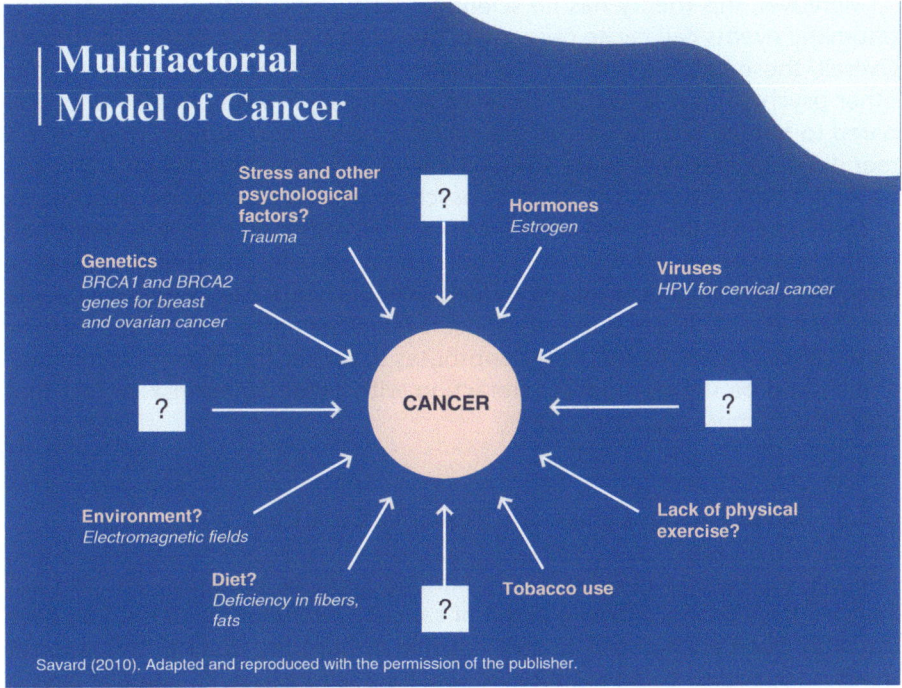

Savard (2010). Adapted and reproduced with the permission of the publisher.

5.2.2 Does Stress Cause Cancer?

It is not simple, if not impossible, to determine the specific causes of cancer. Because they find it hard to deal with such uncertainty, many patients tend to continue searching for the cause of their disease. In the absence of an identifiable medical cause, they will end up concluding that their cancer must have a psychological cause, such as stress. This tendency to conclude that psychological causes are involved when there are no identifiable biological causes for a health condition is not new. For example, for decades, stomach ulcers were believed to be caused by stress until researchers discovered that most stomach ulcers are caused by a type of bacteria that can be treated effectively with antibiotics.

The belief that stress causes cancer is widespread. Indeed, it is not uncommon to hear people say things like: "No wonder he has cancer, he is always under so much stress." Many people with cancer tend to wonder whether stress or a specific event could have triggered their illness. This belief is fuelled by hundreds of pop psychology books suggesting that a person is responsible for their cancer because of their mental attitude. Many people are drawn to this theory because it gives them a sense of control. However, this theory also has its downsides because it generates strong feelings of guilt (*"It is my fault if I have cancer because I did not manage to keep my stress under control"*). It is common for people to feel guilty about having developed cancer. Guilt is a very unpleasant feeling that can lead to depression.

Moreover, this theory has no scientific basis. The hypothesis that stress or traumatic events can cause cancer has been the subject of dozens of studies. Overall, these studies failed to establish a clear link between stress (or any other psychological factor) and cancer. When people with cancer were compared to people who never had the disease, researchers noticed that the former did not experience more stressful events than the latter. When a link was observed between stress or another psychological factor (trauma, depression, or certain personality traits) and cancer incidence, it could mostly be explained by the fact that people who were under stress generally had more unhealthy lifestyle habits, such as smoking. Indeed, lifestyle habits play a clear role in the development of cancer. Currently, most researchers agree that if stress (or any other psychological factor) truly contributes to cancer, its influence is minimal, and should be understood as interacting with other cancer risk factors that play a much more significant role.

5.2.3 Does Thought Have the Power to Cure Cancer?

Another widespread belief is that a fighting spirit or a positive attitude can increase the chances of being cured of cancer. Since your diagnosis, you have probably been encouraged to stay positive to fight the disease. This popular belief is supported by a multitude of books on self-healing. The idea of having power over cancer can seem very appealing, especially in a society that highly values personal control. And since medical research has little information to offer on the factors that may explain a more favourable course of the disease, this leaves room for all kinds of speculation.

Supporters of the power of thought approach tend to cite isolated cases to support their theory. For example, they may describe the case of a man with a fighting spirit who survived cancer despite being told he only had a few months left to live. Or the case of a woman with an extremely negative attitude who, despite an excellent prognosis, had several recurrences that ultimately led to her death. However, our experience as clinical psychologists has shown us that there are definitely as many patients with a positive attitude and a fighting spirit who experience an unfavourable cancer course as there are patients who experience the opposite. Likewise, not all our patients with a negative attitude have seen their cancer progress. In short, we should only give little credibility to theories that are based solely on specific clinical cases because they are subject to bias (such as only reporting cases that confirm said theories) and they do not take

5.2 Can Thoughts Influence Cancer?

into account the whole picture. Scientific research is our only means for rigorously verifying the validity of a theory. Many studies have been conducted to assess whether a fighting attitude or other psychological factors like stress or depression can influence cancer progression. In general, these studies show that a person's mental attitude or psychological symptoms do not have a crucial role.

In 1989, American psychiatrist David Spiegel published a study that related to the belief that mental attitude plays a role in cancer recovery. It was conducted with women with metastatic breast cancer (advanced cancer with no chances of being cured), half of whom participated in group psychotherapy once a week for a year while the other half did not. At the end of the study, researchers observed that participation in the psychotherapy group was associated with reduced psychological distress, including anxiety and depressive symptoms. However, their most remarkable observation was that women who received the psychological intervention lived about twice longer than women who did not, for an average of 37 months versus 19 months. From that point on, the media began spreading the message that psychotherapy could cure cancer and that mental attitude could help beat the disease. However, researchers generally received these results with caution because, in research, a phenomenon must be observed in more than one study before we can conclude that it is real. Indeed, a given research result must be found repeatedly in several studies conducted by different research teams, a process called replication. Thus, researchers stressed the importance of replicating Spiegel's results in other studies. Many replication studies have since been carried out, including one by Canadian researcher Pamela Goodwin, which comprised a larger number of participants (Goodwin et al., 2001). Therefore, it was more rigorous, and its results showed a decrease in psychological distress at the end of psychotherapy, especially in women who had higher levels of distress at the start of the study. However, no difference was found between the groups concerning survival. We will not discuss all the other replication studies published on this topic; in brief, none to this day have successfully replicated Spiegel's initial results.

In short, though some people with cancer defy their doctor's prognosis by surviving much longer than expected, the power of thought or mental attitude has nothing to do with it. Establishing a prognosis is still a very approximate medical act, so it is often inaccurate. Therefore, in the same way that it is difficult to determine why a particular person developed cancer based on the available scientific evidence, it is also hard to explain why some people with cancer experience a more favourable trajectory with the disease than do others.

Why do we feel the need to discuss the validity of these two beliefs? The answer is simply because scientific literature reveals that strongly believing that stress causes cancer or that mental attitude plays a determining role in its progression is associated with higher levels of psychological distress, namely with higher levels of anxiety, depression, and fear of recurrence. Nonetheless, it is recognized that psychological difficulties such as depression and anxiety affect quality of life. Therefore, it is essential to help people who hold such beliefs cope better with their disease.

5.2.4 Can Positive Thinking Help You Cope with Cancer?

As we have just seen, mental attitude does not seem to be linked to cancer recovery. But could it be associated with a better adjustment to cancer? Most studies have focused on the effects of optimism, which is a personality characteristic that changes little over a lifetime, rather than on the thoughts we have daily. Dispositional optimism is the tendency to expect that more positive than negative events will occur in life. The results of some studies have shown that optimism is associated with experiencing less psychological distress in the context of cancer.

However, there is a growing body of scientific evidence that calls for caution regarding unrealistic optimism. In a study conducted with patients with Parkinson's disease (Hurt et al., 2012), researchers observed that optimistic patients were less depressed at the time of their diagnosis. However, when their disease had progressed, patients who were initially more optimistic had higher levels of depression compared to patients who had initially reacted more negatively.

In other words, having what could be described as unrealistic optimism at the time of diagnosis, such as thinking that the disease is not that serious, may offer psychological protection in the short term, but in the long term, it can impair adjustment to the illness, for example when it progresses.

5.3 The Cognitive Model of Emotions

5.3.1 Cancer: A Distressing Experience

Being diagnosed with cancer is a distressing experience. The word "cancer" alone has a strong emotional connotation. Many negative thoughts are likely to occur after receiving a cancer diagnosis, such as: "I am going to die" (indeed, cancer is still often associated with death despite survival rates that improve every year), "I am going to suffer and so will my loved ones," "This is unfair!" or "It is my fault." The cancer experience can also trigger several negative emotions such as sadness, anxiety, guilt, anger, and so on. Of course, it also comes with daunting challenges and many people must undergo numerous treatments that involve several unpleasant side effects. Most patients will have to stop working for a while, which can lead to financial concerns. However, the factor that will have the most influence on a person's psychological reaction is their perception of their situation.

The idea that our perceptions are crucial in determining the nature and intensity of our emotional reactions stems from the cognitive-behavioural approach, a school of thought that emerged in the early 1960s. Although several authors have developed models of their own, we mainly refer to the principles of cognitive therapy elaborated by Dr Aaron T. Beck, a psychiatrist associated with the University of Pennsylvania in the United States. Many scientific studies have shown that cognitive therapy is an effective treatment for various psychological disorders, including depression and other mood disorders, anxiety disorders, and other conditions involving a psychological component such as chronic pain,

5.3 The Cognitive Model of Emotions

chronic fatigue syndrome, and insomnia (Chaloult, 2008). Further, cognitive-behavioural therapy, a broader class of psychotherapies that includes cognitive therapy, is among the most scientifically supported psychotherapies for reducing psychological distress associated with cancer (Compas et al., 1998).

Now that we know this approach is based on scientific evidence, we shall explain the underlying theory of cognitive therapy. Our reactions to events vary based on the type of thoughts we have, whether negative, positive, or realistic. The cognitive model of emotions goes a little further in its explanation by proposing that it is not the event as such that triggers reactions such as sadness, anger, or anxiety, but rather how we interpret it. There are several different ways to react to the same event. Hence, it is the situation as we perceive it, not the situation per se, that determines the nature and intensity of our emotional reactions.

The following figure illustrates the cognitive model of emotions developed by Dr Beck, which clearly shows that our thoughts determine our reactions. Our thoughts and beliefs are part of a broader category called "cognitions," hence the name of the approach and theoretical model. Cognitions that emerge spontaneously in our mind while in a certain situation are called automatic thoughts because of their sudden nature. Brief and impactful, they come to mind without warning. Automatic thoughts are often repetitive, which means that we often tend to have the same kinds of thoughts and reactions when faced with the same type of event. Furthermore, although automatic thoughts are often incorrect or irrational, they still feel true to us. Finally, as indicated in the model, negative reactions are not purely emotional: they can also be behavioural and physiological.

The cognitive model of emotions

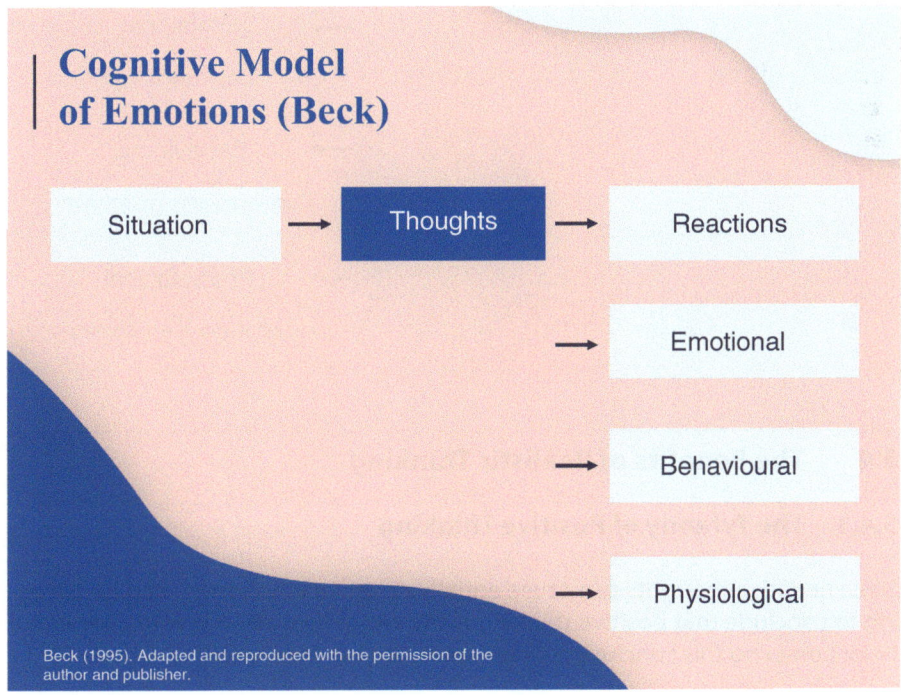

Beck (1995). Adapted and reproduced with the permission of the author and publisher.

5.3.2 The Cognitive Model and Adjustment to Cancer

You may be wondering how all this applies to cancer. The answer is quite simple: as with any other stressor, your reaction to cancer will mainly be determined by your interpretation of it.

Therefore, you will feel anger if you tell yourself that life is unfair (*"Why me?"*), guilt if you blame yourself for developing your disease (*"It is my fault if I have cancer because I did not take enough care of my health"*), helplessness if you believe that you have no control over what happens to you (*"There is nothing I can do about this situation"*), or sadness and anxiety if you are convinced that the outcome of your cancer is fatal (*"I am going to die"*). Since we tend to have more than one type of thought about the same event, we often experience a combination of emotions as a result.

The cognitive model of emotions and cancer

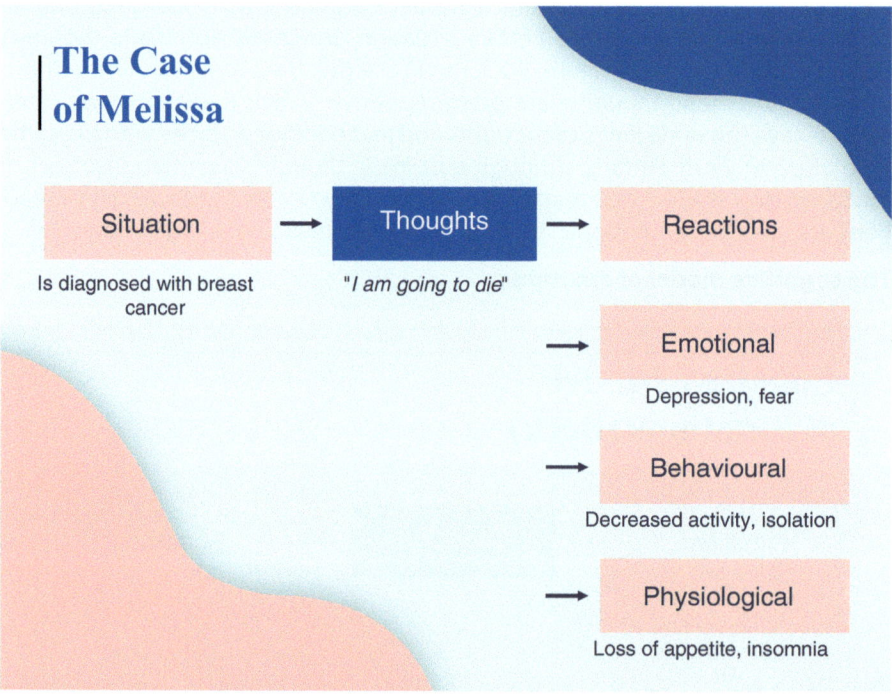

5.4 The Benefits of Realistic Thinking

5.4.1 The Tyranny of Positive Thinking

Since negative thoughts can cause equally negative emotions, it can be tempting to conclude that positive thinking is the key to living better with cancer. But before drawing this conclusion, let us take a look at Jane case:

5.4 The Benefits of Realistic Thinking

> Jane is being treated for breast cancer. She often feels sad and anxious about her prognosis. Having read several books on the power of thought, she is convinced that her sadness and anxiety will harm her chances of being cured. She feels guilty about not managing to maintain a positive attitude ("I am unable to stay positive. So, this cancer will surely kill me"). She decides to see a psychologist in order to improve her chances of recovery.

As this example illustrates, the "tyranny of positive thinking" (Holland & Lewis, 2000) [1] can stir up many negative emotions, namely, strong feelings of guilt, because it is impossible for a person who has just been diagnosed with cancer and who is fearing for their life to remain positive all the time. Cancer is a serious disease that has many consequences on a person's life. Therefore, it is normal to feel afraid, sad, or even angry. As shown in this example, the more Jane tries to stay positive, the less she manages to do so and the more anxious and guilty she feels. The following figure illustrates the vicious circle of positive thinking.

The vicious circle of positive thinking

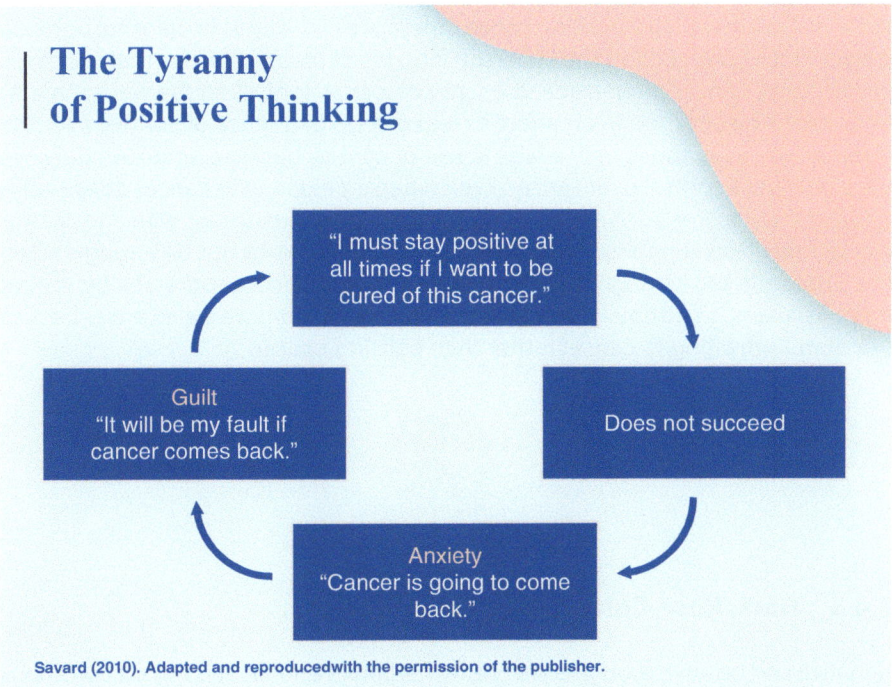

Savard (2010). Adapted and reproduced with the permission of the publisher.

Moreover, when you try to think positively ("This cancer will not get the best of me!" "I will get better," "Having cancer is a good thing, I will learn from it"), you

---

[1] Expression used by Dr. Jimmie Holland, M.D., who is considered as the pioneer of psycho-oncology, a field of research and practice that focuses on the psychological aspects of cancer.

may temporarily succeed in blocking negative emotional reactions. However, this effect will only be short-lived. Like a boomerang, negative thoughts tend to come back with as much, if not more force ("I am going to die," "This will be my last Christmas," "I am no good for anything anymore"). Why? Because positive thoughts are often difficult to believe! Sooner or later, you will begin to doubt your positive thoughts and revert to negative thoughts that are associated with negative emotions such as sadness and anxiety. This perpetual inner battle between positive and negative thoughts demands a lot of energy over time and the latter, which are much more powerful, often end up taking over.

In short, the positive thinking approach has two major drawbacks: it tends to make people feel guilty when they do not manage to remain positive at all times (so, basically everyone!), and the emotional relief it provides does not last over time.

5.4.2 Fighting Cancer?

The positive thinking approach often advocates the warrior metaphor according to which one must fight cancer. However, this idea can also make people with cancer feel deeply guilty because where there is a fight, there is a winner, but there is also a loser. This "fighting cancer" metaphor is likely to be harmful because it puts a lot of pressure on the ill person who is not responsible for their disease's progression. Cancer often leads to a sense of loss of control, so the warrior metaphor might be adopted in an effort to regain a certain sense of control over the disease. However, this is only a false sense of control because, unfortunately, we have only little control over cancer. Even when a person with cancer does everything in their power, such as following the prescribed treatment plan and changing certain lifestyle habits (e.g. quitting smoking), it might not be enough when the disease is too strong. Blaming people whose cancer progresses by seeing them as losers is extremely unfortunate. For this reason, we believe it is best to talk about adjusting to cancer rather than fighting cancer.

5.4.3 Dark, Rose-Coloured, or Clear Glasses?

Negative and positive thoughts are not two separate entities. It is this dichotomous perception that often makes people oscillate between the two. A situation may lead us to have negative thoughts that cause all kinds of negative emotions as though we were seeing it through dark glasses. To reduce any discomfort caused by such thoughts, we may try to replace them with more positive thoughts, or if we refer to the glasses' analogy, we may try to replace our dark glasses with rose-coloured glasses. Then, since it is hard to believe these positive thoughts, the only alternative is to revert to our initial negative thoughts, which are very emotionally upsetting.

Dark Glasses vs. Rose-Coloured Glasses

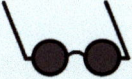

Negative thoughts

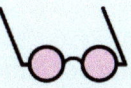

Positive thoughts

Seeing the negative side of the situation
Cancer = death

Seeing the positive side of the situation
Having cancer is a good thing after all; I will learn from this experience

Thinking that everything will go wrong
I am going to die from this cancer

Thinking that everything will be fine
I will be cured of this cancer

In reality, negative thoughts and positive thoughts are each located at the two extremes of the same continuum, which means that they are distributed along the same continuous line.

Realistic Thoughts or Clear Glasses

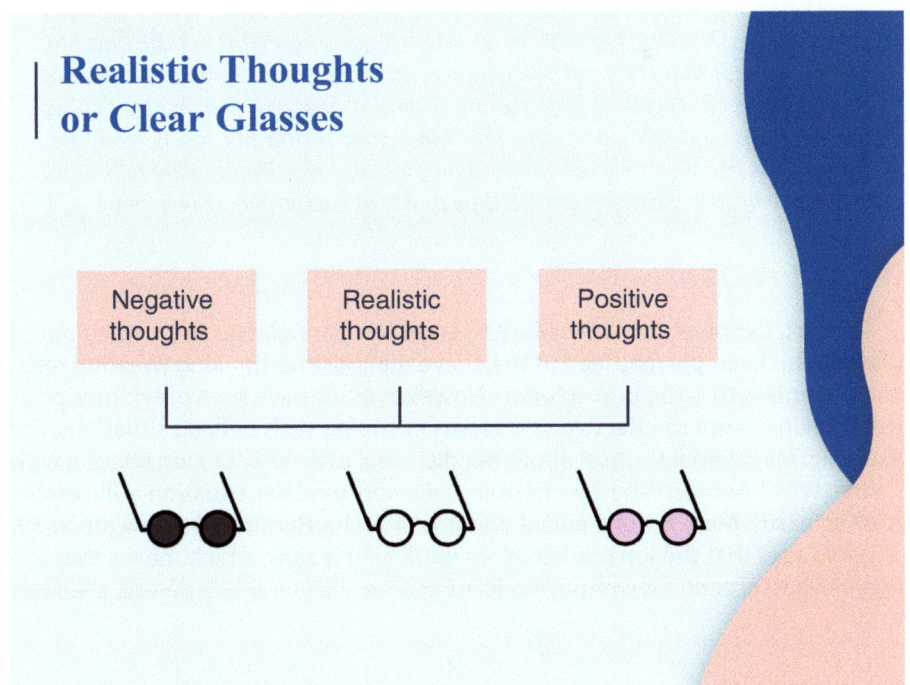

Therefore, there is an alternative to these two extremes, located right in the middle of the continuum: It is called realistic thinking. Using the glasses' analogy, we could say that realistic thinking is like wearing clear glasses. Realistic thinking involves seeing a situation as it is, with both its negative and positive sides. Let us illustrate this with an example that is unrelated to cancer.

> *Mary just found out that she lost her job after 15 years of loyal service. Her reaction to this bad news is very intense as she wonders what she did wrong to deserve such unfair treatment and even thinks that her bosses are very ungrateful to treat her this way after so many years. She wonders whether she will manage to find another job and is afraid that unemployment benefits will have financial consequences on her and her family. "We are headed straight for bankruptcy!"*

Mary is quite negative about her situation as if seeing it through dark glasses. She feels frustrated and betrayed by her bosses, doubts her ability to find a new job, and imagines the worst concerning the impacts of her dismissal on her family's financial security. She does not see any positive aspects of her situation and sees herself as totally incapable of dealing with it.

> *The very day of her dismissal, Mary calls her friend Celine to tell her about what just happened. To cheer her up, Celine tries to get Mary to see the positive side of things by telling her that her situation is good news rather than bad. She points out that Mary has not been happy with her job for a long time and that she now has an excellent opportunity to find a new one that better fits her expectations and skills. She also tells Mary that losing her job is really her bosses' loss because they are losing a model employee. Finally, she tells Mary that she will find another job in no time and that everything will be fine.*

In short, Celine encourages Mary to swap her dark glasses for rose-coloured glasses. This example may lead us to believe that positive thinking (wearing rose-coloured glasses) is the best solution. However, as we have seen previously, positive thinking is not as effective as it seems in coping with difficult situations. For example, Mary remains upset about her dismissal even after talking about it with Celine. Why? Because she has trouble believing that her situation will resolve itself so easily. Mary is quite aware that it is often harder to find a new job at 50. She also sees that the job market in her work field is slow, which means that she may have to accept a lower-paying job. Because she is a single parent, she feels that her fears concerning her family's financial security are legitimate. Therefore, after her conversation with Celine, Mary quickly resumed wearing her dark glasses and her negative thoughts returned. This is precisely the main problem with rose-coloured glasses: it is hard to believe these positive thoughts, so we tend to quickly revert to our negative thoughts. An exhausting mental battle then ensues where negative thoughts are replaced by positive thoughts, and the latter soon end up giving way to the same negative thoughts we had in the first place.

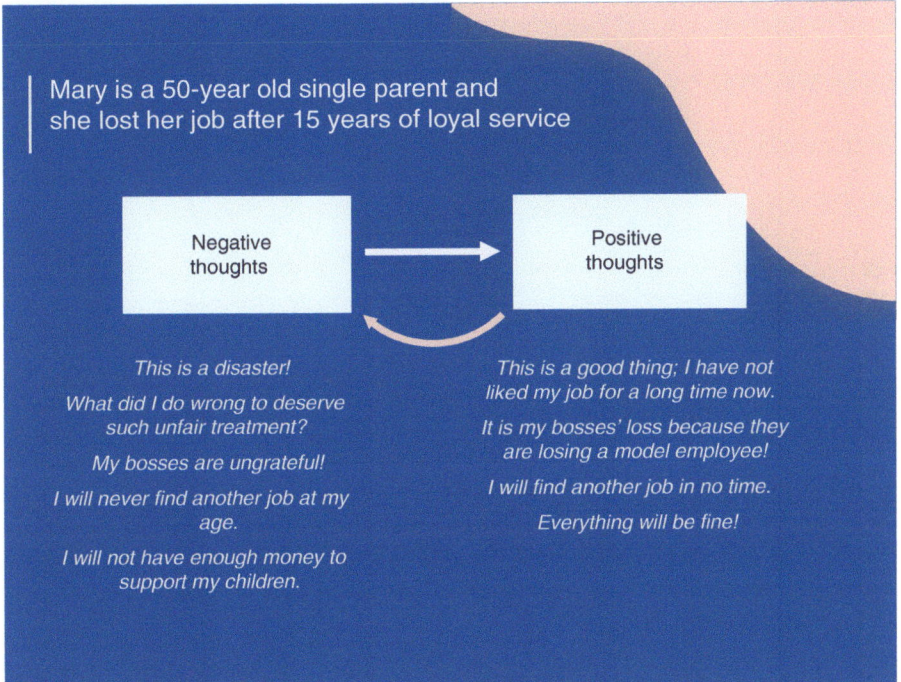

Realistic thinking offers an effective alternative. Through clear glasses or by adopting a more realistic outlook, Mary might see that her situation is very disappointing and frustrating (ideally, she would have preferred to keep her job until retirement), but she could also see it as a challenge ("I can overcome this difficulty"). She might also recognize that it may be more difficult to find another job at her age according to statistics while also identifying her personal strengths and the value of her work experience, which could increase her chances of finding a new job. She might recognize the threat that her dismissal poses to her family's financial security while also knowing that she will be on unemployment benefits for a while, that she will likely find another job in the meantime, and that if worse comes to worst, she could always accept a job that is less suited to her expertise and expectations as a temporary solution and borrow money from her sister.

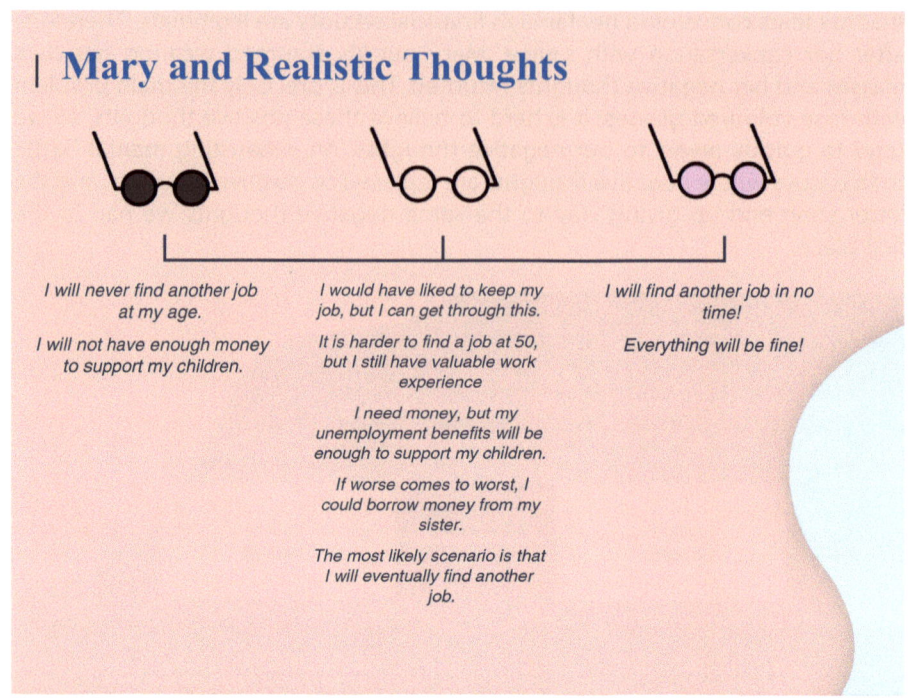

As this example illustrates, realistic thinking helps break the deadlock caused by the constant alternation between positive and negative thoughts. It helps us see a situation in a more nuanced way by considering both its positive and negative sides. It also helps us maintain hope for a favourable outcome that remains realistic. Now, let us see how realistic thinking can be applied to better cope with fear of cancer recurrence.

5.4.4 Realistic Thinking and Cancer

> *Louise has just completed her treatment for ovarian cancer. Because her disease was detected by chance at an early stage, her prognosis is excellent. Her oncologist even told her that she has a 95% chance of recovery. Despite this, Louise is sure that her cancer will come back and that she will die from it, which would ultimately deprive her children of their mother. Louise feels anxious, depressed, and discouraged.*

Obviously, Louise sees her situation through dark glasses. She does not seem to grasp that her chances of recovery are much higher than those of having a cancer recurrence. She even seems to believe that if she had a cancer recurrence, it would necessarily be fatal. One of the possible solutions that could help Louise feel better is to resort to positive thinking. She might then try to convince herself that a recurrence cannot occur in her case. Indeed, she has always had good luck in life, so why would that change now? Louise could also tell herself that she will very surely see her children grow up, as well as her future grandchildren. Once again, though this approach is very appealing (who does not like stories that end well?), it is quite likely that Louise will not truly believe these positive thoughts, or she will only believe them for a short while until the negative thoughts come back just as strong, if not stronger. Why? Because sooner or later, Louise will inevitably question this overly optimistic view of her future and realize that not all hardships happen only to others. Indeed, how is she so special that nothing bad could ever happen to her?

But is hope not essential when living with cancer? Of course, the answer to this question is yes! However, to maintain hope, it is not necessary nor even desirable to wear rose-coloured glasses. You just need to wear clear glasses and see reality as it is without magnifying its negative aspects or adopting an outlook of blind optimism. This approach could also be called "realistic optimism," which involves seeing the real risks of a situation along with its different possible scenarios, all while hoping for the best. As we will see in this program, it is also the most effective way to cope with cancer and reduce fear of recurrence! Here is how Louise could change her negative and positive thoughts into more optimistic and realistic ones.

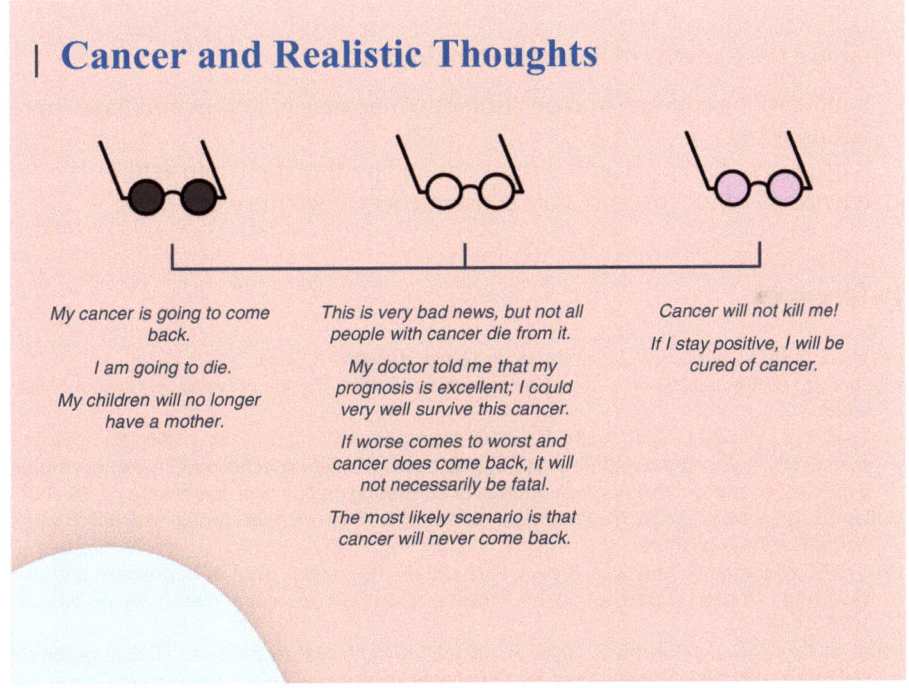

Cancer and Realistic Thoughts

My cancer is going to come back.
I am going to die.
My children will no longer have a mother.

This is very bad news, but not all people with cancer die from it.
My doctor told me that my prognosis is excellent; I could very well survive this cancer.
If worse comes to worst and cancer does come back, it will not necessarily be fatal.
The most likely scenario is that cancer will never come back.

Cancer will not kill me!
If I stay positive, I will be cured of cancer.

At this point, you may be wondering whether it would be relevant to adopt the realistic thinking approach to help you cope better with cancer and reduce your fear of recurrence. If you tend to experience emotional roller coasters and your mood tends to alternate between states of happiness and gloom, it is probably because you are caught in a mental battle between negative and positive thoughts. In this case, realistic thinking could be a good option for you.

In Summary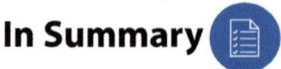

What Is Realistic Thinking?

- It is seeing a situation as it is.
- It is seeing all the possible aspects of a situation without exaggerating them negatively (negative thoughts) or positively (positive thoughts).
- It is seeing all the possible realistic scenarios, all the real risks of a situation, while still hoping for the best.
- It is maintaining realistic optimism.

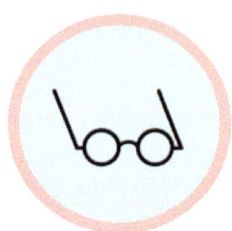

What Are the Benefits of Realistic Thinking?

- It reduces the strength and persistence of negative emotions and has a more lasting effect.
- It helps with finding practical solutions and putting them into action.
- It helps us adjust to all possible consequences, even the worst ones.

References

Beck, J. S. (1995). *Cognitive therapy: Basics and beyond*. Guilford Press.
Chaloult, L. (2008). *La thérapie cognitivo-comportementale: Théorie et pratique*. Gaëtan Morin Éditeur.
Compas, B. E., Haaga, D. A. F., Keefe, F. J., Leitenberg, H., & Williams, D. A. (1998). Sampling of empirically supported psychological treatments from health psychology: Smoking, chronic pain, cancer, and bulimia nervosa. *Journal of Consulting and Clinical Psychology, 66*, 89–112.
Holland, J., & Lewis, S. (2000). *The human side of cancer: Living with hope, coping with uncertainty*. HarperCollins Publishers.
Hurt, C. S., Weinman, J., Lee, R., & Brown, R. G. (2012). The relationship of depression and disease stage to patient perceptions of Parkinson's disease. *Journal of Health Psychology, 17*, 1076–1088.
Lebel, S., Ozakinci, G., Humphris, G., et al. (2016). From normal response to clinical problem: Definition and clinical features of fear of cancer recurrence. *Supportive Care in Cancer, 24*, 3265–3268.
Savard, J. (2010). *Faire face au cancer avec la pensée réaliste*. Montréal: Flammarion Québec.

Session No. 2

6.1 Cognitive Restructuring

In the first session, we explained how negative thoughts cause emotional distress and that positive thinking is not an effective strategy in the long term. We also saw that realistic thinking is an alternative solution that offers more lasting benefits. The first tool that we will present today to help reduce your fear of recurrence is cognitive restructuring, a core technique of cognitive-behavioural therapy. The goal of cognitive restructuring is to question your negative thoughts and turn them into more realistic thoughts.

6.1.1 Cognitive Restructuring

The first step of cognitive restructuring is to identify the automatic thoughts that underlie our negative emotional reactions. This exercise can be challenging because we rarely take the time to notice our thoughts. Filling out a thought record grid (see the grid below) is the most effective way to accomplish this task. Putting this information into writing will allow you to effectively identify the thoughts that underlie your unpleasant emotions, to put into specific words otherwise vague thoughts, especially those we tend to avoid.

The first part of the exercise is to enter the following information into three columns:

1. **Situation:** What situation triggered my negative emotions? When describing the situation, it is crucial to note observable, uninterpreted facts. For example, if someone had witnessed the situation, what would they have seen?
2. **Automatic thoughts:** To fill out this column, the best way to proceed is to ask yourself the following question whenever you experience negative emotions:

Which thought(s) or image(s) came to mind when I felt unpleasant emotions?

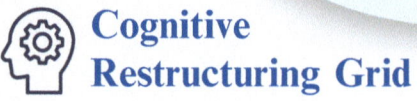
Cognitive Restructuring Grid

Situation	Negative thoughts	Emotions (%)

Beck (1995). Adapted and reproduced with the permission of the author and the publisher.

3. **Emotions:** In this column, note the emotions you felt (e.g. sadness, anxiety, helplessness, anger, etc.). We also suggest that you evaluate the intensity (%) of each emotion you felt, where 100% is the highest intensity. Doing this will eventually help you see if the cognitive restructuring strategy helped reduce the intensity of your negative emotions.

The second step of cognitive restructuring is to question the accuracy and validity of your thoughts using the Socratic questioning method. This step will also help you identify other possible interpretations of the situation and to gain a more realistic perspective. Here is a list of helpful questions to challenge your interpretations:

Key Cognitive Restructuring Questions

- What evidence do I have that this thought is true? Or that it is false?
- Is this thought based on facts or impressions?
- Is there another more likely explanation?
- What is the worst-case scenario, and could I adjust to it? What is the best-case scenario? What is the most likely scenario?
- Is it a question that cannot be answered?
- Is this thought useful? What are its advantages/disadvantages?

Here, we stress the importance of asking yourself what the worst-case scenario would be, even if it is hard or unpleasant to think about it. According to the realistic optimism perspective, it is essential to consider all possible scenarios, even the worst one, and to reflect on how you could adjust to it if it were to occur. Conversely, it is also important to ask yourself what the best-case scenario could be. Finally, identify the most likely and realistic scenario among all the possible ones.

Again, we suggest that you do the exercise in writing. Writing will allow you to take a step back from your initial negative thoughts. Also, writing down realistic thoughts gives them more weight and has a more immediate and significant effect than simply identifying them in your mind. Finally, when the same negative thoughts resurface, you can read what you have already written down and achieve a beneficial effect more quickly since you will not have to repeat the exercise over again from the start. The cognitive restructuring segment of this exercise is carried out by adding two columns to the grid that you used to identify your automatic thoughts:

4. **Realistic thoughts:** Using the key cognitive restructuring questions will help you come up with alternative answers and more realistic thoughts that you may write down in the fourth column. Then, you will begin to see other possible scenarios and determine which one among them is the most likely. Because negative thoughts are often quite powerful, it is usually necessary to find more than one realistic thought to counter the effect of negative thoughts.
5. In the fifth column, you will **reassess the emotions you felt and their intensity** after your interpretation of the situation has changed. If the intensity of your emotions has significantly decreased, it means that cognitive restructuring helped you successfully identify and restructure the negative thoughts that were at the root of your emotion. If your emotions decreased only slightly or not at all, it could mean that certain negative thoughts were not properly identified and restructured. Therefore, it might be necessary to continue to question your negative thoughts to find more realistic and effective alternative thoughts. However, remember that it is normal if your emotions did not completely disappear, especially if you have to deal with a very difficult situation. Often, reducing the intensity of an emotion to a tolerable level is a more realistic goal.

Cognitive Restructuring Grid

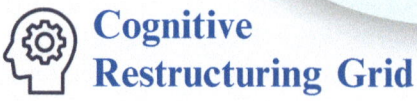

Situation	Negative thoughts	Emotions (%)	Realistic thoughts	Emotions (%)

Beck (1995). Adapted and reproduced with the permission of the author and the publisher.

6.1.2 Cognitive Restructuring and Fear of Cancer Recurrence

> Elise is very anxious about a potential breast cancer recurrence. Each time she experiences a physical symptom, she tends to think that it is due to a cancer recurrence. One day, she was distraught because she had had a headache for a few days and was afraid that it was being caused by brain metastases.

First, let's identify Elise's automatic thoughts and her associated emotions.

Cognitive restructuring grid: The case of Elise

Situation	Negative thoughts	Emotions
"I've had a headache for the past few days."	"I must have brain metastases." "I won't make it through the winter."	Anxious (100 %) Depressed (100 %)

Now, let's see how cognitive restructuring could help Elise reinterpret the situation and reduce her anxiety and depression. Remember that realistic optimism involves considering all possible scenarios, including the worst one, while still hoping for the best. In Elise's case, is there any evidence that her headache could be due to brain metastases? Or conversely, does she have reasons to believe that her headache could be explained by something else? Is there another more likely explanation? What is the worst that could happen? And what is the most likely scenario? The answers to these questions will help Elise develop more realistic alternative thoughts, such as those in the cognitive restructuring grid below. The reassessment of Elise's emotions shows that the exercise effectively reduced her anxiety and depression. Note that the latter are not at 0% even after Elise came up with more realistic thoughts, which leads us to specify that the goal of cognitive restructuring is not to eliminate negative emotions. Cancer and the possibility of recurrence remain sensitive subjects that may still make you feel anxious to a certain degree. Thus, the goal is to reduce negative emotions to a more tolerable level and make them less overwhelming.

Cognitive restructuring grid: The case of Elise

Situation	Negative thoughts	Emotions	Realistic thoughts	Emotions
"I've had a headache for the past few days."	"I must have brain metastases." "I won't make it through the winter."	Anxious (100%) Depressed (100%)	"I usually have this kind of pain a few days a month. It's probably just a normal headache." "My latest test results didn't reveal any signs of cancer." "The more I worry about my headache, the more likely it is to get worse." "If my headache persists or worsens, I will see my doctor to make sure that everything is fine." "The worst that could happen is finding out that I have metastatic cancer. It would be tough news to take; I would be devastated. However, there are treatments for metastases, and I would not necessarily die within the year." "The most likely scenario is that my headaches have nothing to do with cancer."	Anxious (30%) Depressed (20%)

It is important to understand that while cancer recurrence is certainly not desirable, it is not necessarily synonymous with death. There are many different types of recurrence. For example, local recurrences are unlikely to be fatal. Even metastatic recurrences are not necessarily fatal, depending on their site and extent. In all cases, it is relevant (and vital!) to maintain realistic hope about a favourable outcome.

We may not like to think about it, but we are all going to die someday. This is perhaps the only certainty that we have in life. We can illustrate this by seeing ourselves as being on a one-way road leading to death, but many paths can lead us to this outcome. The following figure shows a few possible paths after being diagnosed with cancer. Without a doubt, the worst scenario is being diagnosed with a metastatic recurrence that will rapidly lead to death. Emotionally, this is the most difficult scenario to think about. However, without denying it as a possibility, it is important to remember that many other paths are possible. For example, you could remain in remission from cancer for the rest of your life and die of another cause. You could also develop a local recurrence in a more or less near future and receive another series of treatments and be in remission for a long time after. You could also have a metastatic recurrence in the short, medium, or long term, receive palliative treatment and have a good quality of life for many years before dying from cancer. The goal here is to show you that many different scenarios are possible. Therefore, it would be a shame to consider only one scenario - especially the worst one – and worry about it excessively when there is room to hope for the best possible outcome.

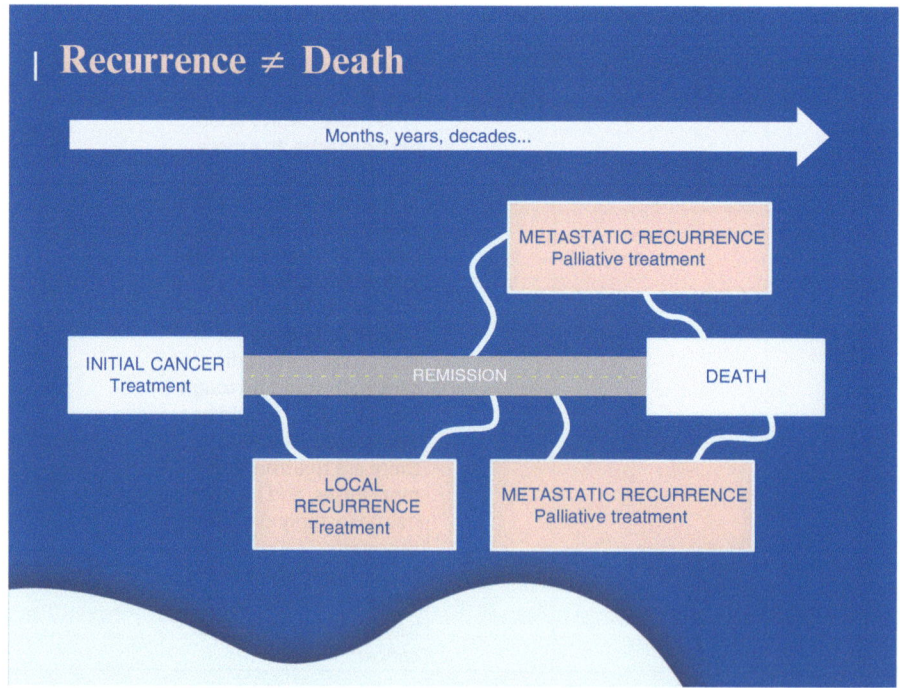

6.2 Interpreting Physical Symptoms Realistically

After being diagnosed with cancer, patients often experience various physical symptoms. They can be due to cancer as such, but they can also be short-term or long-term side effects of treatment, or physical symptoms unrelated to cancer that have been experienced before and are interpreted differently since having cancer. Anxiety can also cause several symptoms (e.g. shortness of breath, stomach aches, etc.). All these symptoms are likely to be interpreted as possible signs of cancer recurrence. After having experienced illness, we often become more mindful of our physical symptoms. For some people, like Elise in the previous example, such monitoring may become chronic. Due to the possibility of cancer spreading to other organs, any unusual symptom is likely to be interpreted as a sign of recurrence.

There are two types of extreme attitudes that people may adopt towards their physical symptoms. On the one hand, there is negligence, which is the tendency not to pay attention to our body at all; this is not necessarily a good thing because we could miss crucial signs of a recurrence or another health problem. It can also be an avoidance strategy that aims to keep our mind off of the disease. Later, we will see that avoidance is not an effective strategy to deal with anxiety. On the other hand, there is hypervigilance, which is the tendency to pay a lot of attention to our physical symptoms and dramatize them or interpret them catastrophically. Such an attitude is likely to increase our anxiety because the more we focus on a physical symptom, the more intense it seems. Hypervigilance is kind of like looking at a symptom through a magnifying glass. To demonstrate this point, do the following exercise: try to recall the sensation of nausea and concentrate very hard on what you feel. We bet that you will probably end up feeling a little sick to your stomach! This is why it is important not to pay more attention than needed to a physical symptom and instead seek a certain balance between attitudes of negligence and hypervigilance, which are both just as harmful as the other.

To achieve a balanced attitude towards your physical symptoms, remember that even people without a history of cancer experience physical sensations daily. They can be pain or other sensations such as digestive troubles, muscle stiffness, and so on. Therefore, it is normal to experience physical symptoms to a certain degree, especially as you age.

To reduce your fear of recurrence, you must learn to interpret your physical symptoms (i.e. internal cues as seen in the fear of cancer recurrence model) realistically. The challenge lies in separating what is normal from what is suspicious, that is to say, what requires medical attention. We suggest using the four following criteria to analyse the physical symptoms you are worried about in a more objective way: **Novelty, Intensity, Likelihood, and Persistence.** You can easily remember them with the following acronym: NILP.

If your symptom is **new** and difficult to explain, and you have never talked to your doctor about it, it is crucial to do so as soon as possible. Conversely, if you have already experienced a given symptom and your oncologist has told you not to worry about it, or if it is not among the signs of recurrence, an immediate consultation is probably unnecessary. You could wait until your routine follow-up to talk about it. For example, Elise had headaches regularly before she had cancer. Her symptom was not new, so it probably did not require an immediate consultation.

Another criterion to consider is symptom **intensity**. For example, Elise could have asked herself the following questions: "Is it a mild headache that will go away within a few hours after taking a Tylenol or Advil tablet?" "Is it a severe headache?" "Is the symptom more frequent or more intense than usual?" If so, we recommend seeing a doctor about it. Moreover, if the symptom is accompanied by other symptoms like nausea, dizziness, or troubled vision, an urgent medical consultation is required.

It is also essential to consider the **likelihood** that a symptom is associated with a cancer recurrence. In Elise's case, while brain metastases can indeed cause headaches, her latest test results came back normal. So, it is rather unlikely that her headache is due to brain metastases. Another example is a person with severe back pain. When they wonder what could have caused this pain, they remember that they were doing gardening the day before. Hence, it is most likely that their back pain is due to gardening rather than cancer recurrence.

The last criterion is symptom **persistence**. This is probably one of the most important criteria to consider when assessing your physical symptoms. A persistent symptom is of greater concern and should be reported to the medical team. Therefore, it is essential to set a time limit after which you will see a doctor and have some tests done if you still have the symptom. As already mentioned, your task is to find a healthy balance between negligence and hypervigilance, which means paying attention to your symptoms without doing so excessively. By giving yourself a little time before seeing a doctor, you could see how your symptom progresses. What makes it worse? What alleviates it? This information will be helpful to health professionals if you decide to seek medical attention. Also, by waiting, you will be faced with the task of tolerating discomfort. Eventually, this approach will help you learn to manage your anxiety about cancer recurrence instead of seeking medical attention repeatedly, as this strategy only provides temporary relief. We will come back to this point later.

In short, the aim is to take a step back from your symptoms to assess them more objectively by using the four criteria (NILP) and make a better, more informed decision about seeking medical attention or not.

6.2.1 Seeking the Right Information on Your Condition

Another element to consider is the level of information you tend to seek about your disease. As we have seen in the fear of cancer recurrence model, this fear is influenced by the degree of knowledge you have about your cancer. However, the level of information required to adjust well to this situation varies from one person to another. Indeed, one person could feel quite comfortable having little knowledge about their condition, while another could find this difficult to bear. Conversely, a patient may become upset if they learn a lot about their disease, its treatment and possible side effects, and their chances of being cured, while another person may feel relieved to know everything. In short, it is up to you to determine whether you know enough about your type of cancer to maximize your psychological well-being. However, it is usually best to avoid extreme attitudes.

People who tend to experience a lot of anxiety (and people who have a high fear of cancer recurrence) may adopt one of the two most extreme information-seeking attitudes. On the one hand, some people want to know as little as possible. If you recognize yourself here, you might not know enough about your condition. Perhaps you have not asked all the questions you are worried about because you are afraid that the answers would upset you even more? As we will see later, this can be a form of avoidance that worsens your anxiety instead of alleviating it. Just because you do not ask your questions to the medical team does not mean that they are not on your mind. Without clear answers from a reliable source, you can still find answers on your own, but they may not be accurate or helpful.

On the other hand, some people want to know everything and seek every bit of information they can find right down to the slightest details. This profile includes various behaviours, such as intensive research on the Internet, regularly participating in discussion forums, asking a lot of questions, sometimes even repeatedly to the different health professionals involved in their care, and seeking information from other people who have also had cancer. The aim of these behaviours is often to regain a certain sense of control over their situation and obtain reassurance. However, when it becomes excessive, this pattern of information-seeking behaviours also tends to maintain anxiety because it exposes the person to more or less reliable and even contradictory information depending on the sources consulted, which creates confusion that may worsen fear of cancer recurrence.

In short, an important step in your journey to reduce this fear is to make sure that you understand your disease well and know your recurrence risk without resorting to excessive information seeking. Having this knowledge will allow you to consider more realistic future scenarios.

6.3   Being Well Informed

In order to better assess the accuracy of your interpretations, it will often be necessary to ask your questions to your treating physician, usually your oncologist, who is a much better source of information than the Internet ("Dr. Google"), your friends, or other people who have been treated for cancer. Indeed, some websites are very unreliable and convey all kinds of inaccurate information. You can still trust certain websites, such as those of official cancer organizations. However, it can still be challenging to find information on your specific type of cancer, even on reliable websites, because each form of cancer has its own characteristics. It is possible to read something and think that it concerns you when this is not necessarily the case, thus creating unnecessary confusion and anxiety. Moreover, although your friends and support groups can be a significant source of support, your doctor remains the only person who knows everything about your particular case. Your friends and other acquaintances do not necessarily have the required medical knowledge or the overall picture of your medical condition to be in a position to judge what applies to you.

In this regard, it can be helpful to prepare a list of questions before attending your medical appointments to avoid forgetting to ask any of them. Referring to this list during your medical consultation will allow your doctor to see how important these questions are to you, which will put them in a good position to answer them. However, if your list is very long, there is a good chance that your doctor will not have time to answer them all, so it is essential to target the questions that are most important to you. Nevertheless, you have the right to ask your questions and obtain the information that you need.

Finally, we suggest attending your medical appointments with a relative or a friend. Health professionals often tend to give a lot of information quickly, and it is not always easy to understand their vocabulary (medical jargon is often pretty obscure!). Do not be afraid to ask for clarification because they do not always realize that their language can be difficult to understand. It is even more difficult for an anxious person who also has to manage their emotional reactions. Studies reveal that patients retain only 20 to 60% of the information they are given during medical consultations. Therefore, a significant proportion of this information is immediately forgotten. The person accompanying you will have more emotional distance, which will help them better memorize the information given during the consultation. They can even take notes that you could read afterwards in a more relaxed setting. Having someone act as a "secretary" during your medical consultations will allow you to better concentrate on what the doctor has to say to you. This person can also validate your interpretation of the topics discussed during the consultation. Another option – but only if your doctor gives you their authorization first – can be to use a device (or your cell phone) to record the information provided during the consultation so you can listen to it later on. Plus, health professionals are often better communicators when they know they are being recorded!

6.4   Interpreting Probabilities and Statistics

People with cancer often want to know their chances of being cured. Many doctors systematically choose to share this information with their patients by using statistics available in scientific literature. One of the first statistics that may be presented to you is recurrence risk. For example, if you are told that you have a 20% chance of having a cancer recurrence, this means that out of 100 people with a form of cancer similar to yours, 20 will have a cancer recurrence, and 80 will not.

Another statistic you may be told about is the net survival rate, which represents the probability of surviving cancer in the absence of other causes of death. For example, let's say that the relative 5-year survival rate for breast cancer is 87%. This means that in a group of 100 people who were diagnosed with breast cancer, 13 people will have died from their cancer five years after their diagnosis and 87 will still be alive.

Finally, another statistic you may be faced with is the reduction in recurrence risk based on the proposed treatment. For example, you may be told that receiving a particular treatment will reduce your recurrence risk by 50%. It is vital to understand that this statistic is based on your actual recurrence risk. For example, if a person with a recurrence risk of 20% receives a form of treatment that reduces their recurrence risk by 50%, it means that their recurrence risk would decrease from 20% to 10%.

Though the risk of cancer recurrence is never zero, it is important to remain hopeful that you will be among those who will experience a more favourable outcome. However, as we have seen previously, you must have realistic hope and remember that you must also be prepared for other possible scenarios.

There are many things to consider when interpreting cancer-related statistics. First, a statistic is an average that is based on hundreds, even thousands of people. Second, it is essential to interpret the numbers correctly; many people tend to overestimate their recurrence risk. Such was the case for Louise: even if her oncologist had told her that she had a 95% chance of never having a recurrence, Louise was convinced that cancer would come back. It was as if her 5% risk had become 100%. Often, the anxiety experienced by patients about recurrence risk is disproportional to their actual recurrence risk. In such a case, it can help to apply the probability to a happy outcome, such as winning the lottery. What would you think if you were told that you have a 95%, 75%, 50%, or even 30% chance of winning the lottery? We "bet" that you would feel somewhat confident of winning, and with reason! Remember that your chances of winning the lottery can be as low as one in many millions! However, this does not stop people from buying tickets and dreaming about winning the lottery someday! Why not be just as confident when cancer recurrence is concerned? The bottom line is that if you can hope to win the lottery and dream about how you would spend the jackpot with only an infinitesimal chance of winning, then perhaps you can also allow yourself to hope that cancer will not come back, whether your recurrence risk is 90% or 10%. Regardless of the statistic involved in your case, it is always possible (and recommended!) to hope to be part of those who will not experience a recurrence.

Third, statistics used by doctors to establish prognoses are constantly changing. Even the most recently published data are based on patients from previous years. For example, to calculate the relative 5-year survival rate statistic, researchers must conduct analyses on patients diagnosed five years earlier to verify whether they survived within this time frame. For this reason, these statistics may not apply perfectly to your reality because they are not representative of the current state of affairs and do not take into account the continuous improvement of treatment. Keep in mind that the field of oncology progresses rapidly, and better treatments are constantly being developed and used.

Moreover, cancer progression, like its initial occurrence, is influenced by various genetic, hormonal, environmental, and behavioural factors. Therefore, each cancer case is unique and progresses according to its own determinants. Also, for reasons that remain unknown, not everyone responds the same way to the various oncological treatments. This fact reinforces the idea that statistics are not necessarily an accurate reflection of your specific case. Therefore, it would be legitimate for you to hope that your prognosis will be better than predicted while also recognizing that the opposite could be true, too.

In Summary

Key Cognitive Restructuring Questions

- What evidence do I have that this thought is true? Or that it is false?
- Is this thought based on facts or impressions?
- Is there another more likely explanation?
- What is the worst-case scenario, and could I adjust to it? What is the best-case scenario? What is the most likely scenario?
- Is it a question that cannot be answered?
- Is this thought useful? What are its advantages/disadvantages?

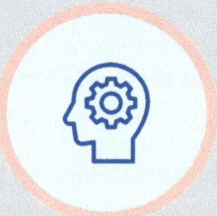

Interpreting Physical Symptoms Realistically (NILP)

- **Novelty:** Is this symptom new?
- **Intensity:** Is this symptom particularly severe or more severe than usual? Are other symptoms present?

- **Likelihood:** Could this symptom be due to something else (e.g. back pain after gardening)?
- **Persistence:** Does the symptom subside after a while? How long should I wait before seeing a doctor?

Being Well Informed

- It is important to seek the amount of information you need and with which you feel comfortable.
- Your doctor and treatment team are the best sources of information for your specific case.
- It can be helpful to prepare your questions before your medical appointments, to be accompanied by someone during these appointments, or to record them (after obtaining the health professional's consent).

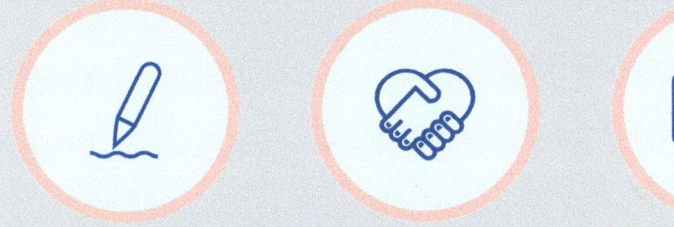

Interpreting Probabilities and Statistics

- Statistics change over time, are based on large numbers of people, and may not accurately represent your specific case.
- It is a good idea to take a step back and put into perspective the statistics related to your case.
- It is possible and recommended to maintain realistic hope no matter what numbers are concerned in your case.

Reference

Beck, J. S. (1995). *Cognitive therapy: Basics and beyond*. Guilford Press.

Session No. 3 7

7.1 Intolerance of Uncertainty

In the previous session, we explained that cognitive restructuring aims to turn negative thoughts into more realistic or "realistically optimistic" ones. This strategy brought us to work on the "Interpretation" box of the fear of cancer recurrence model. This component plays a pivotal role in the onset and maintenance of fear of cancer recurrence. We also discussed how to realistically interpret physical symptoms and statistics and how to seek the right information on your medical condition. Now, we will explain how you can learn to better tolerate uncertainty. Intolerance of uncertainty (illustrated in the background of the model) is a difficulty dealing with not knowing what will happen in the future. Since it is impossible to predict the future ("Will cancer come back or not?"), it is important to become more tolerant of uncertainty to limit any unpleasant emotions that stem from it (e.g. fear, anxiety, hopelessness). Uncertainty is a part of life. For example, while moving to another city for a new job may be a positive event, it still involves a great deal of uncertainty: "Will I find a suitable house for my family? Will I like my new job? Will my children make new friends?" A person who is intolerant of uncertainty, or "allergic" to it, will have more trouble adjusting to this type of situation.

7.2 Learning to Tolerate Uncertainty

Cancer is a disease that involves a great deal of uncertainty. Many people who have been treated for cancer have trouble dealing with such uncertainty. Even for cancers with an excellent prognosis, it is impossible to accurately predict whether a recurrence will occur or not. While many people look forward to making it through a five-year period without any sign of cancer to be considered in remission or even cured, cancer recurrence unfortunately remains a possibility, even after five years. Sometimes, oncologists mention a recurrence risk percentage to their patients, but because the likelihood of being cured is never 100%, this information is not always reassuring, especially for people who are intolerant of uncertainty. When a person is uncomfortable with uncertainty, they tend to be more anxious and try to adopt all sorts of strategies that make them feel like they have more control over what could happen in the future. For example, they may plan excessively for the future, constantly check themselves for signs of recurrence (self-exams), seek reassurance from health professionals, and avoid certain situations that make them feel anxious. However, because it is impossible to plan or control everything, none of these strategies are effective in the long term. Rather than desperately trying to increase your level of certainty about the future, it is best to learn to become more tolerant of uncertainty. An important step toward achieving this goal is to reduce avoidance and reassurance behaviours, which we will discuss further in this manual.

How is it possible to live happily while knowing that cancer could come back at any time? How is it possible to continue to make plans for the future when you do not know whether you will still be there to make them happen? Control is highly valued in Western societies. We like feeling that we have control over our lives. However, we all know that it is impossible to control everything, especially our health. Just as you could not prevent the occurrence of your first cancer, you cannot completely prevent an eventual recurrence. We do not have total control over our health, and the same is true for life in general: life is full of unexpected events and uncertainties. In fact, the only thing we know for sure is that we are all going to die someday. We do not know when or how, but we know that is what lies ahead for us all. And yet, this does not prevent people from being happy.

So how can we be happy without being sure that we are completely cured of cancer? Well, the same way we manage to be happy without being sure that our relationship will last a lifetime, that our children will not become delinquents, that our parents will not develop Alzheimer's disease, or that our house will not be destroyed in a fire. The idea is to focus on the good things that life has to offer rather than on unfortunate events that could occur in the future. Plus, uncertainty is not always a negative thing: the future also has good surprises in store for us!

7.3   Erroneous Beliefs about Worry

To become more tolerant of uncertainty, you must first become aware of your beliefs about worrying because some of them might stand in the way of change. Indeed, it could be more of a challenge to let go of your worries if you believe that they serve a purpose. Here are a few examples of the most common beliefs about the usefulness of worrying. Do you agree with any of them, even partially?

7.3 Erroneous Beliefs about Worry

> **False Beliefs About the Usefulness and Impact of Worrying**
> 1. **Worrying can help solve problems.**
> 2. **Worrying can help prevent negative or unpleasant emotions.**
> 3. **Worrying can influence future events:**
>   - **Worrying can trigger unfortunate events.**
>   - **Worrying can prevent unfortunate events from happening.**

One way to challenge a belief is to examine the evidence that it is true. For example, if you believe that worrying will help you solve a problem, you could list the evidence that shows that this belief is true (*Which issues did I manage to solve by worrying?*) and the counter-evidence that shows that it is false (*Are there problems that I worried about and still did not solve? Have I ever solved problems when I was in a more relaxed, calm, and rational state?*).

Belief :	
Evidence	Counter-evidence

By doing this kind of exercise, you will quickly realize that worrying rarely helps us find solutions to our problems. On the contrary: the more we worry, the more we fret over our problems, which ultimately keeps us from clearly identifying them along with possible solutions. Plus, how can it be useful to spend hours and hours imagining and worrying about various scenarios that might never occur? It is best to live in the present and deal with problems when they arise. The old saying "We will cross that bridge when we come to it" applies perfectly here.

You can also make a list of evidence and counter-evidence for the belief that worrying can help prevent negative emotions (*Has worrying in advance about a problem ever kept me from experiencing unpleasant feelings? Would worrying about an eventual disaster, like the death of my partner or child, protect me from negative emotions if it were to occur?*). As it happens, worrying never protects us from unpleasant feelings. On the contrary, worrying in itself can stir up many unpleasant emotions.

We have already seen that thoughts do not have any power over the occurrence or progression of cancer. Yet, you may have once thought: *"If I worry about cancer recurrence, I will trigger it. I must not think about it."* Conversely, you may also have thought the following: *"If I tell myself that I am cured and let my guard down, cancer will come back."* These two contradictory beliefs have something in common: they both suppose that thoughts or worries have power over events, which is more in the realm of superstition than reality.

The first belief is that worrying about a situation will trigger it. A person who holds this belief will tend to chase away any thoughts about cancer for fear of triggering a recurrence. This strategy is called cognitive avoidance. It can be effective in the short term, but it is often harmful in the long run. Did you really worry in advance about all the unfortunate events that you experienced so far? Or on the contrary, have you experienced hardships that you did not worry about beforehand?

Conversely, the second belief is that worrying is useful, that it reduces the likelihood of something happening, and that it is risky to not worry about cancer recurrence. To challenge this belief, you could once again do the evidence and counter-evidence exercise. Evidence: *What were the situations that I dreaded and that did not happen after all?* Counter-evidence: *What events still took place even after I worried about them? What are the hardships that I did not experience despite not worrying about them?*

You can also try to do another exercise to challenge your beliefs: a behavioural experiment (or reality test) that allows you to verify a belief's basis in reality. If you believe that thinking about an event can trigger it, you could try forcing yourself to think about an unfortunate event for 20 to 30 minutes a day and see whether it occurs. For example, you could worry about catching a cold or about one of your loved ones getting into an accident. This exercise will prove to you that worrying about events does not trigger them.

In short, even if these beliefs are widespread, the proposed exercises will have helped you see that worrying does not directly impact the course of future events. It is important to question these beliefs because if you believe that worrying is useful, you will have trouble learning to worry less. Holding such beliefs allows us to feel in control of our lives, but this is just an illusion. In truth, the future is uncertain, and the only actual control that a person with cancer has is over their way of adjusting to their disease.

7.4 The Importance of Facing Your Fears

Let's go back to the explanatory model of fear of cancer recurrence. The previous sections focused on the realistic interpretation of internal and external cues that may trigger fear of cancer recurrence and the importance of becoming more tolerant of uncertainty. The following sections will focus on the importance of facing situations that make you feel anxious. We will explain how behavioural and cognitive avoidance and seeking reassurance and control can help maintain the vicious circle of fear of cancer recurrence. We will also show you how to reverse this process through gradual exposure to your fears.

7.4 The Importance of Facing Your Fears

We have previously seen that negative thoughts can trigger negative emotions. Some behaviours can also play a pivotal role in how we adjust to our experiences and may even maintain worrying over time. Avoidance is a common strategy used to deal with anxiety, but it is a harmful one. It is a deliberate (voluntary) effort not to face situations or thoughts that cause anxiety or any other negative emotions, such as sadness or guilt. Avoidance provides immediate relief because as soon as we avoid something that we fear or that makes us feel uncomfortable, we feel better. However, avoidance is only effective in the short term and is likely to maintain and even increase anxiety in the long term. This phenomenon is illustrated by the avoidance curve (zigzag line) in the following figure. As an example, let's take a situation unrelated to cancer.

7.4.1 Avoidance and Habituation

Avoidance and habituation curves

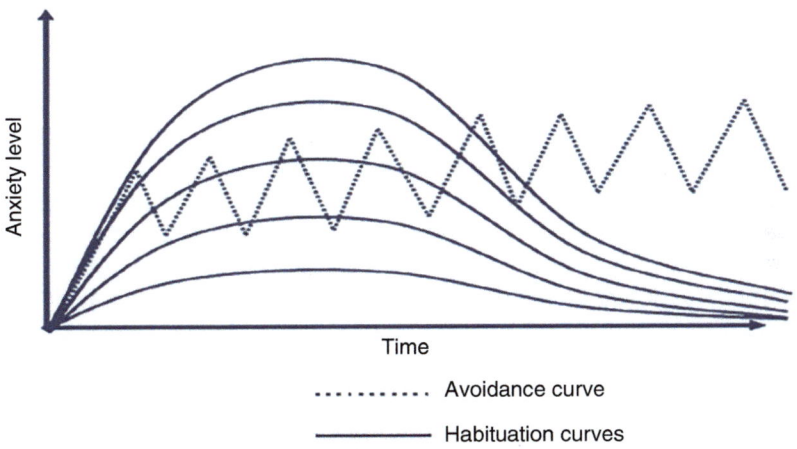

Imagine a person involved in a car accident that turned out to be quite a traumatic experience. This person obviously feels very anxious at the idea of driving their car again and tries to avoid this situation at all costs. When they need to go somewhere, they take public transit. Sometimes, they also decide not to attend a planned activity. Each time they avoid driving their car, their anxiety instantly decreases. Therefore, avoidance is an effective strategy in the short term. The problem is that when the person needs to go somewhere again, their anxiety will be just as high as it was the first time, if not higher. The relief they felt by avoiding the situation they feared somehow confirms that they successfully escaped danger, leading them to believe that avoidance is an effective strategy. However, avoidance will only maintain their fear of the situation. The avoidance curve (zigzag line) shows that driving anxiety will only tend to increase over time.

What would happen if the person instead chose to face their fear? The first time they drive again to go somewhere, their anxiety would be even higher than if they had decided to avoid the situation altogether (see the first habituation curve at the top of the figure). At that moment, they would be extremely uncomfortable. However, their anxiety would eventually decrease because the body cannot remain in such a highly activated state forever. Moreover, their anxiety would decrease more gradually than when they simply chose to avoid driving. Exposure to a feared situation is a particularly beneficial exercise when it is repeated. If the next day, the person decides to overcome their fear by driving again, their anxiety would still rise to a fairly high degree, but not as high as the day before. And if they drive again on Day 3, Day 4, Day 5, and so forth, their anxiety would decrease slightly faster each time. The person would soon notice that by facing the feared situation (in this example, driving their car), their anxiety always decreases a little more each time, and it does not last as long. This phenomenon is called habituation, represented by different curves (continuous lines) in the figure. In addition to the fact that behavioural exposure allows the brain and body to react less strongly to a feared situation, it also helps change our thoughts and beliefs. By driving their car, the person will soon see that nothing unfortunate has happened to them, that they did not get into another accident. This observation will ultimately lead them to challenge their belief that driving is dangerous.

7.5 Behavioural Avoidance and Cancer

This form of avoidance occurs when people seek to flee situations or places associated with cancer. Some examples of behavioural avoidance are: avoiding asking your doctor questions about your disease for fear of the answers you could get, avoiding self-exams of the area of your body that was affected by cancer (e.g. breast, testicle, etc.) for fear of finding a lump, not showing up for medical appointments for fear of signs of recurrence being detected, and avoiding talking about cancer with others and watching television shows or reading books on cancer for fear of triggering uncontrollable worries.

> **List of Common Cancer-Related Avoidance Behaviours**
> - **Avoiding asking questions to your doctor for fear of the answers you could get.**
> - **Avoiding self-exams for fear of finding something abnormal.**
> - **Postponing, delaying, or neglecting medical appointments or check-ups.**
> - **Not talking about cancer with others.**
> - **Avoiding running into certain people for fear of being asked about your cancer.**
> - **Avoiding watching television shows or listening to the radio, reading books or newspaper articles about cancer.**

(continued)

> List of Common Cancer-Related Avoidance Behaviours (continued)
> - **Avoiding reading about your type of cancer (documents given by the medical team, reliable websites).**
> - **Fleeing from hospitals, waiting rooms, blood tests, etc.**
> - **Avoiding reading the obituaries.**
> - **Avoiding attending funerals.**

Understandably, people have a natural tendency to avoid facing what they fear. By doing so, they avoid experiencing emotions that they feel incapable of dealing with or find unpleasant. However, as illustrated previously with the driving example, the effectiveness of this strategy is short-lived. The person may feel relieved at first, but their worries will quickly resurface. Suppose they decide to stop attending their annual follow-up appointments. In that case, they would instantly feel relieved about not having to face a possible scenario where they find out that cancer has come back. However, new worries are quite likely to emerge sooner or later (*What if cancer has come back? Would it be too late to treat it?*). But because it provides immediate relief of anxiety, the person may believe that they successfully avoided danger, so they may want to use this strategy again the next time they feel anxious about the same situation.

The more a person flees situations that make them feel anxious, the less functional they risk becoming in the long run, like in the fear of driving example. Indeed, the more the person avoided driving, the more afraid of driving they became, and so, the more limited their activities became. Avoidance behaviours in a person with cancer are likely to be even more harmful because they may pose a risk to their health. For example, a person who is afraid of needles may refuse to undergo chemotherapy, which could reduce their chances of being cured. Likewise, signs of cancer recurrence may go unnoticed in a person who does not do self-exams, which would ultimately delay the detection of a recurrence and harm treatment effectiveness.

It is also important not to confuse avoidance with distraction. For example, you can decide to talk about something other than cancer with a friend out of pure pleasure. To determine whether a behaviour is rooted in avoidance, you must ask yourself about the reason or intention that motivates it. Do you want to talk about something else because you feel that there is nothing more to say about cancer or because you feel too anxious? Are you doing crossword puzzles because you enjoy this activity or because you want to stop thinking about cancer? The answer to these questions is crucial.

7.6 Behavioural Exposure

If you practise avoidance behaviours, we encourage you to confront your fears gradually through a strategy called behavioural exposure. Some general guidelines must be followed for this technique to be effective. First, it should be done gradually. If we take the fear of driving example, a first step could be to drive on small, less busy roads. Once their anxiety has decreased enough, the person could start driving on avenues and boulevards, then on highways. They could also begin the process by being accompanied by someone first, then start driving alone. Second, behavioural exposure should be repeated (e.g. daily). Back to our example: if the person decides to drive their car on a specific day, and they only drive it again a month later, their brain will not remember how well things went the last time and how their anxiety had eventually decreased. This is because too much time has passed between the two behavioural exposure sessions. Third, behavioural exposure should be done over a prolonged period. For example, if the person drives their car only for a short distance and stops just a few minutes later, their anxiety will not have time to decrease, as illustrated by the habituation curves. Therefore, they will remain stuck on their negative experience and lose the motivation to do it all over again. For this reason, each behavioural exposure session must be long enough to allow anxiety to decrease (i.e. usually at least 30 minutes).

To help you identify a first avoidance behaviour to use in the exercise at the end of this section, indicate how often you avoid these types of situations (i.e. never, sometimes, or often) using the exercise at the end of this chapter. Next, note the percentage of anxiety you would feel if you faced each situation that you avoid at least "sometimes." Finally, rank them in ascending order (i.e. from the one that causes the least anxiety to the one that causes the most anxiety).

Here is the behavioural exposure procedure to follow for the behaviours of your choice, along with an example related to fear of recurrence.

> **Behavioural Exposure Procedure**
> - **List and rank your avoidance behaviours (from the least frightening to the most frightening).**
> - **Choose a first avoidance behaviour (should be associated with some anxiety but to a low level).**
> - **Identify the level of anxiety expected during the upcoming behavioural exposure session (0-100%).**
> - **Identify actions that can be taken to carry out the behavioural exposure task (duration, frequency, accompanied or not, etc.).**
> - **Identify the results of the behavioural exposure task (anxiety level, satisfaction).**
> - **Reassess the level of anxiety felt during the behavioural exposure session.**
> - **Add any other relevant observations (advantages and disadvantages).**
> - **Repeat this procedure until the anxiety felt during the exposure session drops to a minimal level.**
> - **Choose another avoidance behaviour from your list and repeat the behavioural exposure procedure.**

7.6 Behavioural Exposure

Targeted avoidance behaviour: Avoiding reading information on cancer

Behavioural exposure task	Anxiety before (%)	Behavioural exposure actions	Results	Anxiety after (%)	Observations
Reading information on my type of cancer.	70%	Reading for 30 min every day for 7 days. Starting with less stressful sections (e.g. treatment) and finishing with the most stressful ones (e.g. recurrence, metastases). Planning a pleasant activity to do after the session.	Anxiety was high at first, then it decreased.	30%	I felt proud of myself for reading this content. Some of the content I read answered some of my questions about my condition. At the end, I feel more confident because I understand my disease better.

In the example presented above, the person's anxiety decreases considerably. However, if you decide to face a highly feared situation, your anxiety may not decrease as much during the first behavioural exposure sessions, which would be completely normal. It is with practice and repeated exposure to the feared situation that your anxiety will eventually decrease.

In Summary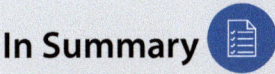

Better Tolerating Uncertainty

- The risk of experiencing fear of cancer recurrence is higher in people who are more intolerant of (or allergic to) uncertainty.
- Instead of trying to increase certainty about the future, it is best to learn to increase our tolerance of uncertainty.
- Uncertainty is not always negative: the future also has good things in store for us.

False Beliefs about Worry

- Worrying can help solve problems.
- Worrying can help prevent negative and unpleasant emotions.
- Worrying can influence future events:
  - Worrying can trigger unfortunate events.
  - Worrying can prevent unfortunate events from happening.

(continued)

In Summary (continued)
How to Challenge These Beliefs:

1. Establish a list of evidence and counter-evidence associated with the belief.
2. Do a behavioural test to verify the basis of the belief.

The Importance of Facing Your Fears

- Avoidance increases and maintains anxiety in the long term.
- Exposure helps us face our fears and reduces anxiety through the habituation process.
- Exposure to the source of fear or anxiety should be:
    - Gradual
    - Repeated
    - Prolonged

Session No. 4

8.1 Cognitive Avoidance

The following sections will focus on another form of avoidance: cognitive avoidance. It occurs when a person tries to keep cancer-related thoughts or images from arising or staying in their mind. A person uses cognitive avoidance when they try to get rid of thoughts about cancer ("No! I can't think about that!"), when they replace such thoughts with other more comforting ones ("Look at how beautiful nature is!"), or when they do an activity with the goal of not thinking about cancer (e.g. watching television, using social media, working, praying, meditating). While this strategy may provide instant relief, it may also increase unpleasant thoughts in the long term. As it happens, cognitive avoidance often leads to the opposite result that is sought when people resort to it. To illustrate this point, we invite you to do the following exercise.[1]

> **The Camel Exercise**
> Close your eyes and try to think about a camel for one minute. Concentrate on thinking only about a camel and nothing else. [...] Then, open your eyes. Was it easy to keep your mind on the image of a camel the whole time? Probably not. You probably thought about other things a few times. If you managed to not think about anything else than a camel, this likely required some effort.

---

[1] The description of this exercise was inspired by Ladouceur et al. (2008), and by Dugas and Robichaud (2007).

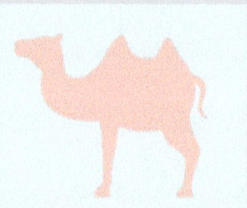

Now, let's try a different exercise. Close your eyes, and this time, try not to think about a camel for one minute. You can think about anything that you want, except a camel. Mentally note the times when the thought or image of a camel popped into your mind despite your efforts not to think about it. [...] Then, open your eyes. Was it hard to avoid thinking about a camel? The answer is most likely yes.

This exercise demonstrates that it is quite difficult to think about just one thing, and even more difficult to force ourselves not to think about something in particular. A camel is usually a harmless subject. However, when an unpleasant emotion is attached to an undesired thought (e.g. fear in response to the idea of a possible cancer recurrence), it is even harder to get rid of the thought. Like behavioural avoidance, cognitive avoidance can provide immediate relief. However, over time, the more you try not to think about cancer, the more you end up focusing on it, paradoxically. Also, it is pretty exhausting for the mind to avoid thinking about something in particular, which ultimately results in a waste of mental energy since this strategy to reduce anxiety is ineffective. Moreover, cognitive avoidance does not help you learn to tolerate unpleasant emotions associated with negative thoughts. To break the vicious circle of avoidance and ultimately reduce your anxiety, we encourage you to face your unpleasant thoughts instead of avoiding them. Here are a few strategies that may help you better deal with unpleasant thoughts.

8.2 Facing Your Thoughts

8.2.1 Cognitive Restructuring

Cognitive restructuring, which was presented in a previous section, is an effective strategy to deal with negative thoughts. Instead of trying to drive away thoughts that make you anxious, you could take the time to identify your negative thoughts and turn them into realistically optimistic thoughts by using the cognitive restructuring technique, that is, by questioning the validity and usefulness of your thoughts and exploring other possible interpretations. Ask yourself questions such as: "What is the evidence that this thought is true?" "Is there another more likely explanation?" "What is the worst that could happen?" A change in perspective could be enough to relieve your anxiety and reduce overwhelming emotions. After all, considering the worst possible scenario is a form of cognitive exposure (see the cognitive exposure description provided further in this chapter). However, if your thoughts keep coming back or catastrophic scenarios persist in your mind, it may be advisable to consider other strategies among those proposed in the following sections.

8.2.2 Planned "Worry Time"

Anxious people tend to worry at different times throughout the day. Because worries often surface at the wrong time (e.g. at work), it is normal to want to drive away disturbing thoughts to reduce their impact on our daily functioning. Planned "worry time" is a strategy that involves determining a convenient moment to deal with troubling thoughts instead of driving them away. To do this, you need to plan a place and fixed time between 5 and 15 minutes during which you will face your worries by letting them surface. This means that if any worries emerge throughout your day, you will have to wait until your planned worry time to examine them. This strategy is different from avoidance because the idea is to face your worries, but later at a predetermined time. This strategy allows you to confront thoughts that cause you anxiety. It also helps you gain some control over these types of thoughts by allowing them to arise at the chosen time while also giving you the opportunity to realize that it is possible to worry without it leading to disaster. Moreover, planned worry time allows you to take a step back from your thoughts, which can help you realize that they are just thoughts, not reality. In the end, you will probably worry a lot less.

8.2.3 Tolerating Unpleasant Thoughts and Emotions

There are other techniques that can help you learn to tolerate thoughts that make you anxious instead of trying to drive them out of your mind. One of those techniques is inspired by the mindfulness approach, which involves placing ourselves as observers of our thoughts. This technique is based on the idea that our thoughts will eventually leave our minds if we give them the chance to do so. When a troubling thought emerges (e.g. *Cancer will come back*), it is crucial not to fight it. Otherwise, the "camel effect" will take place and bring it back with as much force, if not more.

The quicksand analogy can help us illustrate this point. When a person is stuck in quicksand, their natural reaction is to try to escape. By desperately trying to raise one foot to get out of the quicksand, they only put more pressure on the other foot supporting their entire body weight, which only makes them sink deeper into the quicksand. Paradoxically, the only way for the person to escape is to lie down because by increasing the contact area with the mud, the pressure produced by the body decreases, thus giving them the chance to float. In other words, they must stop fighting. The same is true for negative emotions. An emotion is like a wave that comes and goes. You cannot be overwhelmed forever by a feeling: it is just a bad moment that will eventually pass.

In short, it is best to welcome your thoughts and emotions instead of trying to fight them off. Imagine them flowing like water off a duck's back or as clouds that pass through the sky or leaves floating on a river. With practice, you will learn to put your thoughts and their importance into perspective. After all, thoughts are just thoughts, and the emotions they cause can certainly be unpleasant but not dangerous. The idea here is not to make light of your fear of cancer recurrence but rather to help you see that your thoughts are not reality: they are simply a product of your mind.

8.2.4 Cognitive Exposure

Finally, cognitive exposure (or exposure to thoughts) is another effective strategy that can help you learn to face your fears and reduce anxiety associated with fear of cancer recurrence. This strategy is generally used in individual or group psychotherapy, but it is also possible to use it on your own. Cognitive exposure involves imagining a scenario that includes your worst fears and facing them regularly and systematically (by reading the scenario or listening to an audio recording of it repeatedly) until the anxiety experienced becomes tolerable. It may seem counter-intuitive to think about your fears, but just as with behavioural exposure, repeated exposure to catastrophic scenarios leads to habituation. Confronting your most negative thoughts will allow you to get used to them, thus reducing the negative emotions associated with them. Cognitive exposure can also help you realize that although the exercise is unpleasant, nothing bad happens. Confronting your feared scenario in your mind can also help you stop fighting your thoughts, which can provide relief.

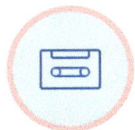 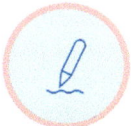

Cognitive exposure is kind of like watching a horror movie over and over again. The first time you watch it, you may experience a lot of fear and disgust. However, if you watch the same movie every day, you will end up noticing that while the horror scenes are still unpleasant to watch, the feelings caused by them are less intense. Therefore, you will be able to take a step back and see that it is just a movie and not reality: it is simply fiction.

To be effective, cognitive exposure sessions must be conducted repeatedly (e.g. several times per week), over a long enough period (i.e. at least 20 minutes), and the scenario must be very detailed (e.g. the specific situation, the people present, the places, the emotions felt, etc.). You can write down your scenario and record it (on your phone, for example) and listen to it over and over again for 20 minutes every day until habituation takes place and your anxiety decreases. It will probably take a while before your anxiety decreases within the session during the first cognitive exposure sessions, but it should subside more and more quickly over the sessions.

The previously described strategies all aim to reduce cognitive avoidance. Among them, you can choose to use those that seem the most suitable to your situation or that work best for you.

8.3 Seeking Reassurance

We have already mentioned that people who tend to worry a lot are often intolerant of uncertainty. To reduce their anxiety, they may try to avoid the uncertainty associated with some situations, such as the possibility of a cancer recurrence. One of the strategies they may use in an attempt to accomplish this is to seek reassurance. For example, a person may try to reassure themselves by thinking that everything will be fine or by asking others to reassure them, such as their loved ones or health professionals. Excessive reassurance seeking usually aims to eliminate all possible doubts about cancer recurrence. However, even with an excellent prognosis, it is impossible to be entirely sure that cancer will never come back or that a new form of cancer will not develop. As with avoidance, seeking reassurance may provide instant relief, but this effect does not last very long because doubts will inevitably resurface.

Reassurance behaviours are another form of avoidance because they keep you from experiencing anxiety about a situation. Seeing a doctor repeatedly to ask them the same questions (*Doctor, am I cured?*), asking to have extra tests run, seeing several health professionals about the same problem, doing excessive self-exams, asking for reassurance from loved ones (*Do you think that I am cured?*), and trying to reassure oneself with ready-made positive thoughts (*Everything will be fine!*) are a few examples of reassurance behaviours that are meant to eliminate uncertainty. It is important to distinguish reassurance behaviours that are excessive from those that are justified. For example, it is normal to seek medical attention for a symptom that meets the objective criteria presented previously (Novelty, Intensity, Likelihood, Probability – NILP). It is also recommended to pay attention to potential signs of cancer progression by conducting occasional self-exams. Also, asking the same questions is not necessarily a problem if you do not remember the answers or if you did not understand them. However, it is a different story when the goal is to hear the same answers over and over again to be reassured or when the person hopes to get a more reassuring answer. It is all a matter of degree and intention. Indeed, if the main reason behind these behaviours is to calm anxiety that is otherwise difficult to relieve (*Only my doctor can reassure me*), and the intensity of these behaviours is excessive (i.e. they overwhelm the person's life and are considered excessive by their loved ones), then it is probably avoidance. It can also help to ask yourself what a person who is less afraid of cancer recurrence would do to determine whether your reassurance behaviours are excessive.

It is important to limit excessive reassurance seeking. While it may reduce your anxiety instantly, you will soon begin to worry again (*What if my doctor is wrong? What if they made a mistake during the test?*). Also, if there are inconsistencies between the things said to you by different health professionals, your anxiety will only increase. Excessive self-checking may also lead to this effect. For example, each time you do a self-exam to make sure that no new lumps or lesions have formed, you will automatically feel reassured. However, doubts will inevitably resurface (*What if I didn't check myself properly? What if a lump has appeared since the last time that I checked myself?*). It is best to learn to tolerate doubt rather than seek certainty that cancer will not come back.

8.4 Seeking Control

Patients commonly wonder what they can do to prevent cancer from coming back, especially during the post-treatment phase. Another widely used strategy to reduce anxiety is to adopt behaviours that help increase their sense of control over the disease, such as changing their diet, exercising more, and practicing visualization. Of course, if these behaviours aim to improve your overall health, daily well-being, and quality of life, they are indeed good lifestyle habits that offer many benefits. However, if they aim to eliminate anxiety about the possibility of cancer coming back, they become part of an avoidance strategy that helps maintain anxiety. Since it is impossible to achieve a total sense of control over cancer, you may end up adopting excessive and rigid goals and feel guilty when you do not manage to achieve them (e.g. I have to walk for one hour every day and not eat any junk food, or else cancer will come back). By setting such high goals that are difficult or even impossible to reach, you will always feel that you are not doing enough to get better. Fear of recurrence then becomes an obsession, a constant worry that can considerably affect your quality of life.

The bottom line is that no lifestyle can eliminate the risk of cancer recurrence. The nutritional organizations' main recommendations are to eat a balanced diet (a lot of fruits, vegetables, and fibre), stop smoking, maintain a healthy weight, and reduce a sedentary lifestyle by being physically active. However, there are no specific standards to reach, so make any changes that you want and feel able to make to feel the best you can and have the best possible quality of life while still enjoying life.

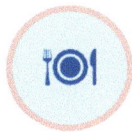  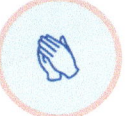

8.5   What If Cancer Comes Back?

For some patients, especially those whose disease is at an earlier stage, the cancer experience will be limited to a single series of oncological treatments. If your tumour was well located and did not spread to other parts of your body, then it is legitimate and realistic to hope that the same scenario could happen again if cancer were to come back.

It is vital to remember that cancer can evolve in many different ways. Some people may have a recurrence in the months or years after finishing their treatment. A cancer recurrence can be local or locoregional (i.e. limited to the tumour's original site or extending only to the immediate surrounding area), or metastatic (i.e. the cancer cells have spread to other areas of the body and have formed masses in other organs, such as the brain, liver, or bones). The type of recurrence will significantly influence the prognosis. Other people may develop a second type of cancer that is unrelated to their first one, and their prognosis will vary depending on the stage at which it was discovered. Again, here is the figure that illustrates the different possible courses of cancer.

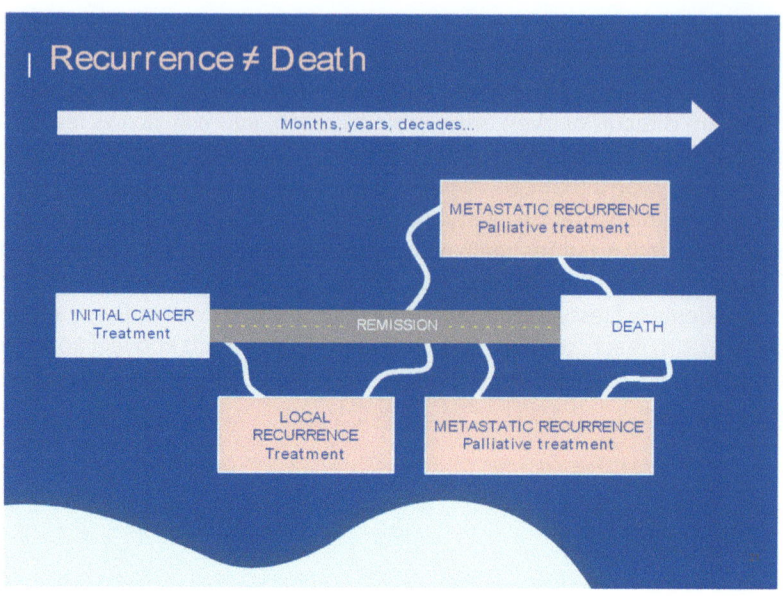

From the beginning, we have insisted that avoidance is harmful and that it is best to face your situation with a realistic outlook. This involves considering all possible future scenarios, including the worst one. Therefore, whether a person's prognosis is good or not, they should consider the possibility of a cancer recurrence head-on rather than trying not to think about this possibility (which would be a form of cognitive avoidance). Of course, it can be upsetting at first to think about such a pessimistic scenario. Still, this strategy will be more effective in the long term because it will allow you to better assess your ability to face such a scenario, contrarily to avoidance that will only cause occasional surges in anxiety that can be very difficult to manage. Being told that cancer has come back is never good news, but recurrences are not always metastatic or fatal. Even if cancer were to come back, it could very well be a localized or locoregional tumour that lends a good prognosis. And a metastatic recurrence does not necessarily mean that it would be fatal in the short term. More and more patients are receiving treatment that successfully controls the progression of metastases and allows them to live for several years with a good quality of life. Unfortunately, some people will end up dying from cancer. These people will have to learn to cope with the idea of dying in the more or less short term, depending on their prognosis. This scenario is indeed part of the risks inherent to cancer, but it is rarely the most likely one in the short term.

Some people are afraid of cancer coming back because it can be fatal, but also because they do not want to have to go through everything they went through after their first cancer experience. Many are convinced that they would not have the strength to get through it a second time. Indeed, cancer treatments are often trying and cause many side effects. But if you managed to make it through treatment once, you are likely to make it through a second time, even if this would be difficult. Remember the resources that helped you get through cancer the first time (e.g. your personal resources, loved ones, community resources, etc.). These resources are quite likely to be there for you again if cancer were to come back. Perhaps your first cancer experience would even help you better deal with the side effects the second time around.

8.6 Redefining Life Goals

It is common for people with cancer, especially those whose cancer progressed, to give up all their life goals. They feel that there is no point in having dreams anymore because they do not believe that they will ever be able to achieve them. But is this true? Is it possible to still have life goals after being diagnosed with cancer? Even in the long term? Is it realistic to have plans even when your life expectancy is reduced? The answer is definitely yes!

It is entirely possible to continue to have life plans by maintaining an attitude of realistic optimism. All you have to do is give less importance to the certainty of fulfilling them someday. Also, can we ever really be sure that we will be able to make our dreams come true? Do we have any guarantee that we will complete a study program? That we will get a promotion at work and grow our business? That we will meet the woman or man of our dreams and have the relationship that we always wanted? That our children will have their own children and hence make our wish of becoming grandparents come true? The answer is obviously no. Life is filled with uncertainty, and we are far from being sure that we will accomplish our goals and fulfil our dreams, even if we lived to be 100 years old. All sorts of events can occur and prevent us from achieving our goals. We are all aware of this reality, yet this does not stop us from making plans, doing what it takes to fulfil them, and having fun along the way. Having plans for the future helps us enjoy life in the present. It gives us reasons to get up in the morning and live our lives. You do not need to be sure that your plans will come to fruition to enjoy the benefits of having life plans and goals. Besides, what is the worst that could happen? We may not have time to complete all of our projects, but we will at least have taken great satisfaction in going through the various towards their achievement.

You may also have to redefine some life goals that are no longer realistic due to your disease. The first step is to examine your past goals. What were your life plans before you had cancer? What were they when you were younger? Did you have goals in the past that you ended up letting go of over time? Did you have dreams that you were not able to fulfil? If cancer had never occurred in your life, what would you want to do? Do not censor your ideas and write down all those that come to mind as if you had no constraints. In the left-hand column of the grid below, write down all your dreams and goals.

Unconstrained goals "magic wand"	Current objectives

Next, in the right-hand column, write down the plans in the left-hand column that are still realistic today. Depending on your current situation, some goals may need to be modified to be achievable. For example, if you dreamed of going on a solo trip to Europe, but your current physical capacities or financial resources are limited, you could readjust this plan by changing its duration and its form, for example, by turning it into an organized, two-week trip to Europe. Likewise, if one of your old dreams was to buy a cabin by a lake, you could instead rent a cabin for the whole summer if you do not have the financial means to buy one. It is definitely much better to readjust old, unfulfilled plans and enjoy life than give them up entirely and live with regrets.

Next, move on to the second step of redefining your life goals, which is to finalize your list of goals and break them down into goals for the short, medium, and long term.

My new life goals	Short-term goals	Medium-term goals	Long-term goals

8.6 Redefining Life Goals

In the left-hand column, write down the goals you identified in the right-hand column of the previous grid that are still important to you. You can also add new goals, such as those that appeared more recently due to cancer. We suggest that you identify goals that are consistent with your core values and that have meaning for you. For a bit of inspiration, you can also ask yourself the following questions:

- **What is truly important to me?**
- **What do I hold dear to my heart?**
- **How do I want to spend the rest of my time on this earth?**
- **How do I want to be toward myself and others?**
- **What qualities do I want to develop?**

Indeed, projects do not have to "cost" anything: they can also be actions that will help you better enjoy life and grow as a person. The goals that you wrote down in the left-hand column will become your new life goals.

Once your list of new life goals is complete, you will be ready to break them down into short, medium, and long-term goals. When do you want to carry out these projects? Which ones are a priority for you right now and should be in the short-term goals column? Also, you may want to break down more complex goals into smaller goals. For example, if you wish to get closer to your grandchildren, you could plan to invite them over for dinner more often (short term), have them over for a whole week during the summer holiday (medium term), and plan to move to the same city as them (long term).

It is important to note that the time frame for each type of goal can vary from one person to another. For example, a six-month period may represent a short-term goal for one person and a long-term goal for another, depending on their perspective and life expectancy. Remember that the primary purpose of redefining your life goals is to give yourself reasons to live each day and enjoy the activities that are meant to help you achieve your goals. The important thing is not to achieve your goals at all costs but rather to have realistic expectations. For example, you could very well aim to get a degree in a particular field if you tell yourself that the most important thing is not to be sure that you will finish the program, but rather to feel satisfaction and a sense of accomplishment for having taken and passed the courses.

Finally, you should go over the previous exercise again from time to time. This will allow you to see how well you have accomplished certain goals and review your plans as your health and physical abilities change. Also, remember that there is no predetermined end to the plans you make: they can remain realistic even if they go beyond the prognosis you are given.

In Summary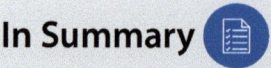

The Importance of Facing Your Thoughts

- Cognitive avoidance helps increase and maintain anxiety in the long term ("the camel effect").
- Many strategies can help you learn to face your thoughts:

    - Cognitive restructuring
    - Planned "worry time"
    - Tolerating negative thoughts and emotions (welcoming them rather than fighting them)
    - Cognitive exposure

Reassurance: A Form of Avoidance

- It is better to learn to tolerate uncertainty than to seek reassurance.
- Reassurance behaviours can be excessive and help maintain anxiety.

A False Sense of Control

- Some behaviours may help increase your sense of control over the disease:
    - Dietary changes
    - Physical exercise
    - Visualization

- Beware of rigid and extreme rules because they cause feelings of guilt and maintain anxiety (impossible to control everything).
- It is best to make changes that are realistic and that aim to improve your general quality of life.

What If Cancer Comes Back?

- Cancer recurrence is not always metastatic or fatal in the short term.
- You have made it through treatment once, so you would likely make it through a second time.
- It helps to maintain goals for the short, medium, and long terms, regardless of your prognosis.

8.7 Conclusion

We sincerely hope that this program and document have been helpful to you. This program undoubtedly helped you better understand the factors that contribute to your fear of cancer recurrence. It may also have helped you realize that you are intolerant of uncertainty and identify specific avoidance, reassurance, and control behaviours that you tend to adopt to avoid feeling anxious. However, bear in mind that while a good understanding of what happens to you is essential, it is rarely enough to reduce anxiety. Now, it is time for you to take action to change certain behaviours, attitudes, and beliefs that maintain your fear of recurrence. We encourage you to take a step further in your personal process to reduce your fear of cancer recurrence. Doing this will probably require a lot of effort on your part, but you will realize that it is well worth it when you start seeing your anxiety decrease gradually. However, this short program may not have been enough to help significantly reduce your fear of recurrence. After a few weeks, if it remains difficult to put into practice the suggested strategies, if you do not manage to make the necessary changes, or if you remain anxious about cancer recurrence so much that it affects your quality of life, it would be advisable to seek individual counselling with a mental health practitioner, such as a psychologist. Furthermore, if you need more support to make the desired changes, we strongly encourage you to talk to your nurse or doctor as they can direct you to the appropriate resources.

References

Dugas, M., & Robichaud, M. (2007). *Cognitive-behavioral treatment for generalized anxiety disorder*. Routledge.

Ladouceur, R., Bélanger, L., & Léger, É. (2008). *Arrêtez de vous faire du souci pour tout et pour rien*. Odile Jacob.

Appendix

Exercise

Identification of negative thoughts about cancer

Situation	Automatic thoughts	Emotions

Which thoughts or images came to mind _____ when you felt the emotion? in the situation _____

Appendix

Exercise

Cognitive restructuring of negative thoughts related to cancer

Situation	Negative thoughts	Emotions (%)	Realistic thoughts	Emotions (%)

Questioning the Validity of Your Thoughts
- What evidence do I have that this thought is true? Or that it is false?
- Is this thought based on facts or impressions?
- Is there another more likely explanation?
- What is the worst-case scenario, and could I adjust to it? What is the best-case scenario? What is the most likely scenario?
- Is it a question that cannot be answered?
- Is this thought useful? What are its advantages/disadvantages?

Exercise

List of Cancer-Related Avoidance Behaviours

For each avoidance behaviour, please indicate:
- How often it occurs (never, sometimes, often).
- How anxious you feel at the idea of facing each of these situations (0-100%). In the last column, rank the behaviours that you sometimes or often avoid from the least scary to the scariest.

Appendix

Behaviours	Never	Sometimes	Often	Anxiety (%)	Order
Avoiding asking questions to your doctor for fear of receiving answers that make you feel anxious	●	●	●		
Avoiding checking yourself for fear of finding something abnormal	●	●	●		
Delaying, postponing, or neglecting medical follow-up appointments or check-ups	●	●	●		
Avoiding talking about cancer with others	●	●	●		
Avoiding running into certain people for fear of being asked about your cancer	●	●	●		
Avoiding seeing or listening to other people with cancer	●	●	●		
Avoiding watching television shows, listening to the radio, or reading books or newspaper articles about cancer	●	●	●		
Avoiding reading about your type of cancer (documentation provided by the medical team, reliable websites)	●	●	●		
Avoiding hospitals, waiting rooms, blood tests, etc.	●	●	●		
Avoiding reading the obituaries	●	●	●		
Avoiding going to funerals	●	●	●		
Other(s): _____					

Behavioural exposure to an avoided cancer-related situation
Targeted avoidance behaviour:

Behavioural exposure task	Anxiety before (%)	Behavioural exposure actions	Results	Anxiety after (%)	Observations

Behavioural Exposure Procedure
- Choose an avoidance behaviour.
- Identify the level of anxiety expected during the upcoming behavioural exposure session (0-100%).
- Identify actions that can be taken to carry out the behavioural exposure task (duration, frequency, accompanied or not, etc.).
- Identify the results of the behavioural exposure task (anxiety level, satisfaction).
- Reassess the level of anxiety felt (during the behavioural exposure session).
- Add any other relevant observations (advantages and disadvantages).

Exercise

Redefining life goals (step 1)

Current objectives

Unconstrained goals "magic wand"

Appendix

Redefining life goals (step 2)

My new life goals	Short-term goals	Medium-term goals	Long-term goals

A Few Inspiring Questions:
- What is truly important to me? What do I hold dear to my heart?
- How do I want to spend the time I have left on this earth?
- How do I want to be toward myself, others, and the world around me?
- Which personal qualities do I want to develop?

Index

A
Anxiety, 6, 7, 12, 13, 15, 26, 28, 31, 35–37, 58, 59, 62, 67–69, 71, 79, 82, 83, 85, 88–92, 105, 110, 111, 113, 117, 120–128, 130–136, 139, 144, 149, 151, 152, 158–165, 181, 185–188, 191–196, 204, 206, 208–211, 213, 217, 221–226, 228–232, 234, 238, 239, 243, 244
Automatic thoughts, 59, 61, 193, 203, 205, 206
Avoidance, 10, 12, 13, 15, 71, 82, 87, 88, 105, 106, 110, 114, 121–132, 134–136, 139, 141, 144, 145, 149–151, 153, 155, 157–161, 163–165, 180, 188, 209, 211, 218, 220–229, 231, 232, 234, 238, 239, 243, 244
  behavioural avoidance, 222, 223
  cognitive avoidance, 227, 228
  and habituation curves, 159, 221, 222
Avoidance behaviour, 87, 105, 106, 121, 124, 131, 132, 134, 222–225, 242–244

B
Behavioural avoidance, 122, 131, 13, 105, 106, 123, 128, 139, 150, 188, 222–223, 228
Behavioural exposure, 106, 116, 122, 123, 126–128, 130, 132–137, 139, 142–144, 157, 222–225, 230, 243, 244

C
Canadian Cancer Society, 134

Cancer, 4–38, 40–44, 49, 54–59, 62, 64, 71, 74, 75, 77–82, 84, 85, 87–94, 97, 98, 100, 105, 107, 110–117, 119, 121–123, 125–132, 134–137, 139–142, 144, 145, 148, 149, 151, 153, 154, 157, 159–171, 173–177, 181, 185–197, 200–203, 206–213, 217, 218, 220–223, 225, 227, 228, 230–235, 237–239, 241–243
Cancer recurrence, 4–6, 8–11, 28, 55, 56, 62, 64, 71, 74, 80–82, 84, 91, 92, 97, 100, 105, 110, 112, 113, 117, 121, 123, 125, 130, 136, 139, 140, 142, 144, 145, 151, 153, 154, 157, 159, 161, 162, 164, 165, 167, 169, 181, 185–188, 200, 206–213, 217, 218, 220, 223, 225, 227, 228, 230–234, 238, 239
Clinical cases *vs.* scientific research, 19
Cognitions, 193
Cognitive avoidance, 13, 121, 123, 139, 141, 144–151, 155, 159, 180, 188, 220, 227, 228, 231, 234, 238
  camel exercise, 145
Cognitive-behavioural therapy, 6, 10, 57–59, 203
Cognitive exposure, 151, 152, 157–159, 180, 229–231, 238
Cognitive model of emotions, 30–32, 192–194
Cognitive restructuring, 60, 62, 67–69, 72–81, 98–102, 107–109, 139, 151, 152, 180, 203–208, 214, 217, 228–229, 238, 242
  automatic thoughts, 203
  emotions, 204
  and fear of cancer recurrence, 206, 207

Cognitive restructuring (*cont.*)
  realistic thoughts, 205
  situation, 203
Cognitive restructuring grid, 72, 75, 98, 99, 107, 108, 205–207
Cognitive restructuring technique, 72, 73, 79, 229
Control behaviours, 239

D
Danish population study, 21
Diet, 23, 24, 140, 164–166, 232, 233

E
Emotions, 8, 12, 13, 15, 26, 27, 30–32, 39, 52, 58, 61, 62, 70–75, 78, 79, 99, 100, 102, 108, 110, 117, 119, 123, 144, 148, 150, 152, 154–157, 159, 160, 173, 174, 186–188, 192–196, 202–207, 217, 219, 221, 223, 225, 228–231, 238, 241, 242
  and unpleasant thoughts, 229
Environment, 23, 40, 213
Excessive reassurance, 139, 159, 161, 163, 231, 232
Explanatory model, 186–188, 220

F
Fear of cancer recurrence, 4–6, 8–11, 28, 62, 71, 81, 100, 105, 110, 112, 123, 144, 145, 151, 154, 161, 164, 181, 185–188, 200, 206, 209–211, 217, 220, 225, 230, 239
  defined, 185
  explanatory model of, 187, 188
  power of thought approach, 190
  psychological factors, 188
  stress, 189
Fear of recurrence, 4, 5, 7, 10–13, 15, 25, 29, 47, 55, 57, 64, 71, 74, 82, 83, 86, 87, 102, 110, 112, 123, 137, 142, 144, 160, 163, 167, 181, 185–188, 191, 201, 203, 209, 224, 233, 239
  characteristics, 10
  factors, 10
  psychotherapy group on, 5, 6
  vicious circle of, 10, 12, 15

G
Genetics, 23

Group interventions, 5

H
Health professionals, 56, 87, 90, 111, 114, 161, 162, 181, 210–212, 214, 218, 231, 232
Hormones, 23, 82
Hypervigilance, 67, 81–84, 209, 210

I
Information-seeking profiles, 86, 107
Intensity, 9, 22, 30, 32, 55, 61, 62, 81, 83–85, 100, 108, 139, 159, 162, 186, 192, 193, 204, 205, 209, 211, 214, 232
Intervention model, 6
Intolerance of uncertainty, 10, 14, 105, 110–116, 123, 137, 139, 142, 144, 160, 185, 188, 217

L
Life goals, 8, 140–142, 170–180, 235–238, 244
Likelihood, 9, 12, 16, 81, 83, 84, 162, 209, 210, 214, 218, 220, 232

M
Mental attitude, 17, 18, 25–29, 40, 43, 190–192
Mental health practitioner, 239
Multifactorial Model of Cancer, 3, 20, 23–25, 64, 165, 189

N
Negative emotions, 13, 31–33, 39, 52, 61, 73, 79, 100, 117, 119, 124, 155, 188, 192, 194–196, 202–204, 206, 219, 221, 230
Negative thoughts, 4, 9, 10, 30, 31, 33, 37–40, 44–51, 55, 57, 59–62, 64, 67, 69, 72–79, 98–100, 105, 107–109, 139, 149–154, 173, 174, 180, 192, 194–197, 199–207, 217, 221, 228–230, 238, 241, 242
  characteristics of, 60
  cognitive restructuring of, 99, 100
  and emotions, 154
  identification of, 61
Novelty, 81, 83, 84, 162, 209, 214, 232

Index

O
Optimism, 3, 8, 40, 47, 50, 64, 67, 69, 77, 91, 140, 167, 175, 192, 201, 202, 204, 206, 235
  dispositional optimism, 41

P
Persistence, 52, 58, 81, 83, 84, 162, 202, 209, 210, 214
Physical exercise, 24, 140, 164, 166, 238
Physical sensations, 82, 83, 186, 187, 209
Positive thinking, 20, 29, 33–43, 47, 49–52, 64, 79, 192, 194–196, 198, 200, 203
  effects of, 38
  vs. negative thoughts, 38
Positive thoughts, 25–30, 37–39, 44, 47, 49, 57, 64, 69, 196, 197, 199, 201, 202, 232
Psychological cause, 23, 189
Psychological factors, 10, 14–23, 25, 29, 188–191
Psychotherapy group, 5–6, 26, 59, 140, 181, 191

R
Realistic interpretation, 68, 92, 107, 220
Realistic optimism, 41, 47, 50, 64, 67, 69, 77, 140, 167, 175, 192, 201, 204, 206, 235
Realistic thinking, 6, 9, 10, 44–57, 64, 69, 175, 194–203
Realistic thoughts, 46, 52, 55–56, 78, 79, 99, 108, 109, 174, 203–207
Reassurance, 13, 88, 111, 114, 144, 159–164, 180, 188, 211, 218, 220, 231–232, 238, 239
Reassurance behaviours, 161–162, 218, 231, 232, 238
Reassurance-seeking behaviours, 162, 163
Recurrence risk, 92, 93, 95–97, 113, 116, 211–213, 218

S
Sadness, 13, 31, 35, 62, 124, 187, 192–196, 204, 221
Scientific research, 19–20, 191
Seeking control, 88, 113, 140, 163–166, 180, 232–233
Sociodemographic characteristics, 186
Spiegel, David, 26, 27, 191
Statistics, 91–98, 107, 199, 212–213, 215, 217
Stomach ulcers, 20, 21, 23, 189

T
Thought identification exercise, 61–62, 70, 71
Tobacco use, 23

U
Uncertainty, 14, 79, 110–116, 142, 161, 162, 180, 185, 186, 188, 189, 217, 218, 220, 225, 231, 232, 235, 238, 239
Unpleasant thoughts, 150, 151, 154, 156, 228–230
  and emotions, 154
Usefulness of worrying, 118, 119, 218

V
Viruses, 24

W
Worrying, 115, 117–119, 121, 122, 137, 151, 185, 218–221, 225
  impact of, 218–220

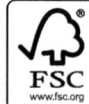

MIX
Papier aus verantwortungsvollen Quellen
Paper from responsible sources
FSC® C105338

If you have any concerns about our products,
you can contact us on
ProductSafety@springernature.com

In case Publisher is established outside the EU,
the EU authorized representative is:
**Springer Nature Customer Service Center GmbH
Europaplatz 3, 69115 Heidelberg, Germany**

Printed by Libri Plureos GmbH
in Hamburg, Germany